Gender, Work and Tourism

M. Thea Sinclair is Senior Lecturer in Economics and Director of the Tourism Research Centre at the University of Kent.

Gender, Work and Tourism

Edited by M. Thea Sinclair

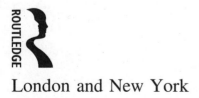

London and New York

First published 1997
by Routledge
11 New Fetter Lane, London EC4P 4EE

Simultaneously published in the USA and Canada
by Routledge
29 West 35th Street, New York, NY 10001

Typeset in Times by
J&L Composition Ltd, Filey, North Yorkshire
Printed and bound in Great Britain by Redwood Books,
Trowbridge, Wiltshire

British Library Cataloguing in Publication Data
A catalogue record for this book is available from the British Library

Library of Congress Cataloging in Publication Data
A catalogue record for this book has been requested

ISBN 0-415-10985-X (hbk)
    0-415-10986-8 (pbk)

Contents

Figures

Tables

Notes on contributors

Sylvia Chant is Reader in Geography at the London School of Economics.

Sara L. Kindon is Lecturer in Regional and Development Studies in the Department of Geography, Victoria University of Wellington, New Zealand.

Veronica II. Long is Teaching Assistant in Geography at the University of Waterloo, Canada.

Margaret Marshment is Senior Lecturer in Media and Cultural Studies at Liverpool John Moores University.

Hisae Muroi is Lecturer in English in the Department of Business and Communication, Bunri College, Tokyo.

Kate Purcell is Principal Research Fellow at the Institute for Employment Research, University of Warwick.

Naoko Sasaki is Research Officer at Global System, Tokyo.

Julie Scott is Lecturer in the School of Tourism, University of the Eastern Mediterranean, Northern Cyprus.

M. Thea Sinclair is Senior Lecturer in Economics at the University of Kent at Canterbury.

Chapter 1

Issues and theories of gender and work in tourism

M. Thea Sinclair

INTRODUCTION

Underlying the images of hedonism and leisure which are commonly associated with tourism is a large amount of work. Holiday-makers engage in tourism to escape from their daily tasks and routines but their leisure and entertainment, along with the services provided for business and special interest tourists, are premised on the labour provided by workers in the tourism industry. The divide between incoming tourists and those working in the industry is particularly acute in many tourist destination areas, where contrasting lifestyles of leisure and work are compounded by considerable differences in income and wealth. The tourism industry is characterized by further divisions between the workers themselves, notably in the form of gender and race. While not as evident as those between tourism consumers and producers, such divisions are significant not only for the operation of tourism but for the relative incomes, status and power of those involved in it. Paradoxically, there has been little attention to these issues to date, the main exceptions being the collections edited by Kinnaird and Hall (1994) and Swain (1995) and a number of individual articles and chapters, particularly in the area of prostitution tourism.

This book aims to contribute to the literature on tourism and gender using a comparative international perspective, integrating the relatively unrelated literatures on tourism, gender and work. The chapters consider a range of tourist locations: the UK, Northern Cyprus, Bali, Mexico, the Philippines and Japan. The studies in the book examine the gendered structure of the tourism workforce in the different international destinations and help to explain the processes which reinforce or challenge gendered patterns of work, gender ideologies and distinctions in income, status, power and control.

The following section of this chapter will discuss a number of issues which have been raised in recent tourism literature and which are related to the theme of gender and work in tourism, notably cultural commoditization, the structuring of work in small tourism businesses and larger firms and the interrelationships between gender, paid and unpaid work. Theories which have been used to explain the gendered structure of the labour force will then be considered in order to provide a context for the studies which are included in the book. The subjects and issues which are examined by each of the authors will be outlined in the final section. The contributions which the authors make to the literature and to an understanding of the gendering of work in tourism will be discussed in the concluding chapter.

GENDER AND TOURISM – RECENT CONTRIBUTIONS

The discussion of gender and work which is included in this section is selective in focusing mainly on recent research, in which the topic has been considered explicitly. The cases considered provide useful examples of the role of gender in work. The discussion uses Swain's definition of gender as 'a system of culturally constructed identities, expressed in ideologies of masculinity and femininity, interacting with socially structured relationships in divisions of labour and leisure, sexuality and power between women and men' (1995: 258). This definition has the advantage not only of providing consistency with previous literature but of signalling the inequalities of work, power and control which gender relations involve.

Work in the tourism sectors of destination areas is concentrated particularly in retailing, accommodation and catering, selling, entertainment and transportation provision. Work involves both material transactions and ideological relations, so that a change in either can involve an alteration of work relations within tourism. The commoditization of culture constitutes a type of production and commercialization which demonstrates ideological as well as material aspects of tourism transactions, involving the transformation of traditional artefacts and practices into commodities which are sold to tourists. As Picard (1993) points out, it is often assumed that tourism impacts on the traditional culture of destinations, strengthening or eroding it in a uni-directional process, while the outcome is, instead, a product of interactions between tourists and local people. Tourists, along with community and governmental organizations, provide material support for particular aspects of local culture so that cultural commoditization has repercussions within the wider political domain (Harrison, 1992; Picard, 1993).

The gender dimensions of cultural commoditization were examined by Swain (1993) in a study of ethnic arts production. Swain showed that most of the Kuna and Sani women who produced handicrafts for tourist markets gained increased power within the household but not within the wider society, where traditional gender roles persisted. The main effect of cultural commoditization appeared to be to counter cultural assimilation, while the responses of individual women to the opportunity to produce for tourist consumption varied significantly. This view is supported by Cone's (1995) detailed study of two Mayan women, one of whom produced handicrafts based on traditional methods and designs, the other providing new craft forms. The first befriended tourists and provided them with increased knowledge of and interactions with traditional Mayan culture. The second, in accordance with her different personal background, identified with tourists and, aided by her earnings from tourism, rejected traditional norms. What both women had in common was the active role which they played in their interactions with tourists and their ability to step outside traditional modes of conduct for Mayan women.

Men can also act as 'cultural brokers' in their relations with tourists although, in Pruitt and LaFont's (1995) study, this occurred within a context in which Jamaican men formed sexual relations with women tourists. The study again raised the issue of the effects of tourism on traditional norms and demonstrated the ways in which power and control are negotiated and can change in new contexts. Women tourists obtain some power by providing men with increased material resources, while men retain much of their power owing to the persistence of many facets of traditional gender roles. The relationships between women tourists and local men generally encounter disapproval from the local community. This is also the case for the Otovaleños in Ecuador, who only accept foreign women into the community if they work hard and conform to local values (Meisch, 1995). In Japan, tourism alters power relations by generating earnings for local people. Holidays based around weaving activities also provide the Japanese women who participate in them with a legitimate purpose for leaving the constraints of their family or paid employment, thereby gaining increased control over their lives (Creighton, 1995).

The provision of accommodation in agro-tourism co-operatives alters prevailing gender norms and enables Greek women to gain increased income and power (Castelberg-Koulma, 1991). Women's work legitimates their access to such public spaces as the village café. However, it is still generally unacceptable for Greek women to frequent coffee houses and tavernas and, elsewhere, it is only some of the younger women who are modifying traditional gender roles by entering bars which cater for tourists from Athens (Moore, 1995). Work in accommodation provision may, in contrast, reinforce prevailing gender norms as in the case of Catalonia and Galicia in Spain, where women's work in catering for tourists who stay on farms is seen as an extension of their domestic roles (García-Ramón et al., 1995). Many women in West Java are responsible for managing small-scale accommodation establishments and also work in such activities as selling food and fruit in the informal sector (Wilkinson and Pratiwi, 1995). Their tourism-induced work load has not been offset by greater help with childcare from their male partners who work as tour guides, in tourist transportation or fish at sea. Employment in relatively large enterprises in the formal sector is dominated by non-locals.

Segmentation in the structure of men's and women's work in tourism also occurs in the diverse tourist destinations of Cornwall, the rest of the UK, the Republic of Ireland, Greece and the Caribbean. Women's work in Cornwall is concentrated in the retailing, hotel and catering sector and tends to be seasonal, part-time and low-paid, although many women have worked in the same tourism establishments for many years (Hennessy, 1994). The majority of the tourism enterprises are owned and managed by outsiders. Work in the UK tourism industry demonstrates considerable flexibility (Bagguley, 1990), although the type of flexible work undertaken is usually related to the worker's gender (Urry, 1990). The characteristics of women's work in retailing and accommodation provision in the Republic of Ireland are very similar to those in Cornwall, with a segmented division of labour within the hotel sector but a lower overall labour force participation rate (Breathnach et al., 1994). Within the formal and informal accommodation sectors in Greece, women undertake the tasks most akin to their domestic labour, such as bed-making and cleaning, for which they receive relatively low pay (Leontidou, 1994). A gendered division of labour also prevails in the accommodation and retailing sectors of the Caribbean, where local men perceive women's participation in servicing activities in the accommodation sector in the context of their domestic caring and mothering role (Momsen, 1994). Western Samoa provides fascinating examples of entrepreneurial roles for women in tourism, including the establishment of hotels, restaurants, handicraft production and retailing, in a context of equal rights of access to family resources for women and men (Fairbairn-Dunlop, 1994). The establishment of a Women's Advisory Committee, supported by a key woman entrepreneur, has resulted in the provision of training for local women, who produce handicrafts for the tourist market. An issue of concern is the extent to which the ethos of production in the context of kin and community needs will change as capitalist work relations are introduced following foreign investment in the accommodation sector.

Gender norms affect both the ways in which labour is supplied within the tourism sector and the nature of the demand for it. Consideration of the demand-side raises the issue of what tourists expect to consume. Urry (1990) argues that consumers envisage the process of purchasing and consumption as involving the provision of a 'social experience' which is conditioned by dominant cultural relations. Consumers' expectations differ in relation to both their gender and that of the employees with whom they interact. According to Broadbridge (1991) in the context of retailing and Adkins (1995) in the context of leisure parks, sexuality is an integral component of social relations. Managers require female employees to dress in a stereotypically feminine fashion and to respond positively to sexual innuendos as part of their interaction with male consumers. Thus, gendered and sexualized modes of behaviour and appearance are often demanded and supplied as part of tourism transactions.

The extreme case of sexualized conduct in tourism is that of prostitution tourism, which has been much discussed by previous authors, for example, Barry (1979), Cohen (1982), Graburn (1983), Truong (1990), Lee (1991), Hall (1992) and Sturdevant and Stoltzfus (1992). Hall (1994) points out that sex tourism results from a range of material factors, including government and foreign interests, and Lee (1991) indicates the ways in which ruling groups in destination countries have supported prostitution tourism. The structure of the sex tourism industry has also evolved according to changes in material circumstances and associated political interests.

Leheny (1995), for example, argues that increasing demand for tourism by Japanese women has played an important role in inducing the Thai government to restrain the most overt manifestations of the sex tourism industry, in an attempt to attract a share of the growing market.

It is clear from the above discussions that women are important producers in the tourism industry and their growing involvement in the paid labour markets of many countries is also increasing their role as tourism consumers. Work in tourism, as in other sectors of the economy, is structured along gender lines and generally conforms to dominant gender norms. A number of explanations of why this is the case will be considered in the following section.

THEORIES OF GENDER AND WORK

Feminist theories which attempt to explain the gendered structure of the workforce differ in terms of both the degree of importance which is attached to capitalism and patriarchy in determining men's and women's role in the workforce and the extent to which the two systems are interrelated. The view that class differences dominate the structure of the labour force is characteristic of the Marxist end of the Marxist–feminist spectrum of analysis. Women's major responsibility for household production and more marginal participation in the paid labour force is said to reduce the cost of reproducing the labour force, thereby permitting employers to lower average wage rates (Himmelweit and Mohun, 1977).

This theory has been subject to the well-known criticisms of failing to explain why women rather than men bear the major responsibility for childcare and domestic labour and radical feminists have argued that it is heterosexuality rather than capitalism which underlies inequality between men and women in the domestic and paid work arenas (Rich, 1983; Raymond, 1986). However, heterosexual relations can only be the root cause of unequal work relations if they incorporate some mechanism whereby men control women's access to paid work and prevent them from retaining a level of income which permits their independent decision-making and survival. It is not evident that heterosexuality, *per se*, incorporates such a mechanism. The concept of male control over women's access to particular occupations is, nevertheless, persuasive and forms the basis of the patriarchal component of the 'dual systems approach'.

Dual systems analysis posits that capitalism creates a hierarchical structure in the paid labour force but is indifferent as to whether men or women occupy specific positions within it. Access to occupations is, instead, determined by patriarchal relations which involve men's control over women's labour, resulting in women's employment in low wage jobs, continued dependence upon men and greater unpaid work within the household (Hartmann, 1979, 1981; Walby, 1986, 1990). Capitalism and patriarchy are, thus, viewed as separate systems within dual systems analysis. Patriarchal relations are also said to predominate within pre-capitalist modes of production when the products of women's unpaid work are sold by men, who retain a considerable proportion, if not all, of the income from them (Delphy, 1977).

Theories which view capitalism and patriarchy not as separate but as interrelated systems (for example, Mies, 1986; Pateman, 1988; Acker, 1990; Cockburn, 1991) may be included within a general approach termed patriarchal capitalism (Adkins, 1995). According to this approach, employers' demand for labour occurs in the context of gendered supplies of male and female labour, producing an occupational hierarchy which is itself gendered in such a way as to further profit maximization. Thus, employers create jobs in a range of occupations which are associated with gendered character- istics and they demand male or female employees who will provide these characteristics. In this way, capitalism takes advantage of prevailing gender definitions, whose origins pre-date the capitalist system of production. Historical analyses of the labour market have provided useful insights into the formation of gender norms, the association of women with the domestic sphere and their exclusion from specific occupations, as in the case of tailoring (Morris, 1986) and printing (Cockburn, 1983). Associations dominated by male workers have, at times, been influential in determining access to work, related wages and skill definitions (Cockburn, 1983; Sinclair, 1991).

Thus, women workers' ability to supply their labour has some- times been constrained by male workers' and employers' power and bargaining arrangements. Research on segmented labour markets (reviewed by Sanfey, 1995) has pointed to the role of trade unions and workplace committees in maintaining divisions between pri- mary and secondary segments of the labour force and the 'insiders' and 'outsiders' who occupy them. Employers pay relatively high wages to retain the skills and experience of (predominantly male) full-time workers in the primary sector, whereas lower wages are paid to workers with lower bargaining power in the secondary sector, where more women are employed (see, for example, Rubery, 1978; Walby, 1988; Crompton and Sanderson, 1990; Rees, 1992). Part-time workers and homeworkers, in particular, have poor wages and conditions of employment.

The patriarchal capitalism approach may be extended to take account of gender divisions between workers who are employed in the same occupations (Adkins, 1995). The inter- and intra-occupational structuring of employment does not result solely from constraints on workers' ability to supply their labour via men's control over women's access to jobs; it also results from employers' and male co-workers' demands that women's and men's appearance and behaviour within the workforce conform to traditional norms and expectations. Such expectations incorporate stereotypical notions of femininity and masculinity which include sexualized relations of production. Sexuality, as a socially constructed concept (see, for example, Swain, 1995), is usually premised on the normality of heterosexual relations and has been argued both to 'contribute to the *production* of economic divisions between men and women' and to be the '*outcome* of the organisation of (gendered) relations of production' (Adkins, 1995: 155). Thus, within a static framework of analysis, definitions of gender and sexuality and labour force divisions are often mutually reinforcing. However, within a dynamic framework, gender and sexuality definitions and labour force divisions may change as the result of external factors. The nature of such changes may be examined in more detail using the concepts of the supply of and demand for different types of labour. Thus, for example, a weakening of patriarchal controls over women's access to particular occupations results in a change in the supply of women's labour, while an increase in expenditure results in an increase in labour demand. Identification of the determinants and relative importance of the supply of and demand for men's and women's labour can shed light on the processes by which the structuring of work is maintained or changes over time.

Analysis of the labour market in terms of labour demand and supply is particularly useful in facilitating a more detailed comparison and evaluation of the different theories which have been put forward to explain the gendered segmentation of the labour force. Production under 'pure' capitalist relations incorporates gender-neutrality in the demand for labour in the context of a gendered labour supply. A patriarchal system of production involves both a gendered demand for labour and control over women's ability to supply their labour, constraints on women's access to work being a key feature of this system. 'Patriarchal capitalism' is characterized by gendering of the demand for labour, on an inter- and intra-occupational basis, in the context of a gendered labour supply. In principle, it is possible for examples of each of these types of production relations to co-exist within a given society, thereby superseding past debates about the relative merits of the different theoretical approaches based on an implicit assumption of exclusivity. The extent to which such co-existence can occur in practice will be illustrated in the case studies included in this book.

Consideration of labour demand and supply is also useful in terms of its implications for action designed to challenge workforce divisions. For example, contexts in which the gendering of the demand for labour appears particularly acute may indicate the need for such measures as equal opportunities or positive action policies. Constraints on women's ability to supply their labour in the paid workforce are often related to dominant ideologies of social sexuality and may alter along with changes in material circumstances. Gender norms differ between different societies and the gendering of the supply of labour varies accordingly. As a particular society is exposed to alternative ideologies and practices, definitions of gender and social sexuality are modified, as are labour market divisions. A key issue is, therefore, to identify the nature of gendering of the demand for and supply of labour, as well as the factors which serve to reinforce or change prevailing definitions and divisions. This issue constitutes a theme which links the chapters in this book.

GENDERED WORK IN TOURISM – KEY ISSUES IN AN INTERNATIONAL CONTEXT

Tourism is a fascinating example of the interaction of differing value systems and of the introduction of material changes via the purchasing power of tourists from outside the destination area. Within this context, gender definitions and the division of labour may be renegotiated. While existing gender definitions exercise an 'independent' influence on the formation of tourism workforce patterns in different areas, the growth of tourism and the social interactions associated with it may modify gender definitions so that, within a dynamic context, gender norms and workforce divisions are, to some degree, dependent on tourism (Swain, 1995). The contributors to this book consider a range of factors which give rise to stability or change in gender definitions, the demand for and supply of women's and men's labour, their income, status and power. The main emphasis is on the gender of those working in and around tourism, rather than of the tourist, and the latter remains an important topic for further research. The chapters shed light on theoretical debates concerning the relevance of capitalist, patriarchal and patriarchal capitalist theories of work. Account is taken of women's access to jobs in tourism and, hence, of the differential supply of men's and women's labour to specific occupations, along with the degree which the demand for labour is structured in accordance with gender and social sexuality. To the extent that labour demand takes account of prevailing gender norms, the differing characteristics of men's and women's labour supply are reinforced and gender divisions in work maintained. However, changes in 'material' variables such as wage rates, or in perceptions of appropriate types of labour, can alter both labour demand and supply and the mutually supportive relationship between gender definitions and labour force divisions, resulting in changes in the structuring of work.

The ways in which gender definitions are formed by tour operators in their brochure depictions of tourists and destination country residents is considered by Margaret Marshment. She takes issue with the argument that women in tourist destinations are generally represented in terms of their sexuality and examines the ways in which class and race, as well as assumptions about household structure, affect the images which tour operators use to market holidays. The role which representations of women in destination countries play in the context of 'exotic holidays' is discussed and depictions of workers are considered in relation to the potential consumers of tourism. Like other contributors to the book, Marshment does not regard women as a homogenous category but takes account of diversity and racial difference.

Kate Purcell's chapter contributes to theoretical debates about the relevance of capitalist, patriarchal capitalist and patriarchal relations of work within the context of employment in the UK hospitality sector. She considers the nature of segmentation of the workforce in different types of tourism and leisure production. Occupations are categorized into contingently gendered jobs, sex-typed occupations and patriarchally prescribed occupations, and the characteristics of each category are examined using a variety of examples from the hospitality sector. Purcell's analysis is relevant to the gendering of the demand for and supply of labour in different types of production relations. The chapter uses empirical evidence to investigate the extent to which women can improve their position in the tourism workforce via increased education.

The gendered structure of work in the accommodation sector is also examined by Julie Scott, in the context of Northern Cyprus. The relative importance of patriarchal and capitalist relations of production in small guesthouses and larger hotels is considered, along with women's and men's roles in production and their social interactions with tourists. Scott considers the role of social sexuality in determining the conditions under which women supply their labour, as well as divisions between women and the designation of alternative gender roles to women of different races. The process by which gender roles are reinforced or changed is examined in the Turkish Cypriot context.

The chapter by Veronica Long and Sara Kindon fills a key gap in the literature on cultural commoditization advanced by Picard (1993), notably on the role of gender. The gendered structure of work in handicraft production, retailing, accommodation and tour provision in Bali is examined, generally in the context of small-scale production. Long and Kindon consider women's role in small enterprises and their social interactions with tourists. They also discuss the degree of participation by men and women in higher levels of decision-making, thereby introducing the issue of the gendering of power and control. Racial differences in the structuring of employment in small businesses and larger hotels are identified. The extent to which tourism is consistent with prevailing gender roles is a key theme of the chapter.

The segmentation of work in tourism in Mexico and the Philippines is examined by Sylvia Chant. Women's work is concentrated in accommodation and catering, selling and prostitution and Chant identifies some of the rationales which underlie the division of work by gender. The processes by which gender definitions are maintained or change are considered in terms of the links between women's paid labour and domestic labour, as well as between paid work and sexuality. Chant examines the relationship between women's work in prostitution, racist stereotypes and material and household circumstances, as well as the effects of changes in women's material position, resulting from their work in tourism, on household structure and on women's and men's status, power and control at the domestic level.

Hisae Muroi and Naoko Sasaki further the literature on tourism and prostitution by analysing changes in sex tourism in the context of shifting material and ideological circumstances. The authors consider the effects on Asian women of campaigns against prostitution tourism in tourist origin and destination countries, combined with the growth of tourism demand by Japanese women. Changes in the composition of prostitution demand between tourist destination and origin countries, and the ways in which women have become akin to commodities which are transported between countries, are examined in the context of gendered and racist stereotypes in Japan. Differences between women from different countries are also considered. The cross-country processes by which women's labour is appropriated and controlled are identified and the role of the law in relation to prostitution is critically evaluated. Muroi and Sasaki consider individual Asian women's experiences and the reasons why they have sometimes resorted to the option of violence. This chapter highlights some of the international interrelationships which are intrinsic to stability or changes in gender definitions in tourism work. The ways in which the authors in this book develop the literature on the issues which have been raised are considered in the final chapter, following the contributions themselves.

REFERENCES

Acker, J. (1990) 'Hierarchies, jobs and bodies: a theory of gendered organizations', *Gender and Society*, 4 (2): 139–58.

Adkins, L. (1995) *Gendered Work. Sexuality, Family and the Labour Market*, Milton Keynes and Philadelphia: Open University Press.

Bagguley, P. (1990) 'Gender and labour flexibility in hotels and catering', *Service Industries Journal*, 10 (4): 737–47.

Barry, K. (1979) *Female Sexual Slavery*, New Jersey: Prentice Hall.

Breathnach, P., Henry, M., Drea, S. and O'Flaherty, M. (1994) 'Gender in Irish tourism employment', in V. Kinnaird and D. Hall (eds) *Gender: A Tourism Analysis*, Chichester: Wiley.

Broadbridge, A. (1991) 'Images and goods: women in retailing', in N. Redclift and M.T. Sinclair (eds) *Working Women. International Perspectives on Labour and Gender Ideology*, London and New York: Routledge.

Castelberg-Koulma, M. (1991) 'Greek women and tourism: women's co-operatives as an alternative form of organization', in N. Redclift and

M.T. Sinclair (eds) *Working Women. International Perspectives on Labour and Gender Ideology*, London and New York: Routledge.

Cockburn, C. (1983) *Brothers: Male Dominance and Technological Change*, London: Pluto.

Cockburn, C. (1991) *In the Way of Women: Men's Resistance to Sex Equality in Organizations*, Basingstoke: Macmillan.

Cohen, E. (1982) 'Thai girls and farang men: the edge of ambiguity', *Annals of Tourism Research*, 9 (3): 403–28.

Cone, C. Abbott (1995) 'Crafting selves: the lives of two Mayan women', *Annals of Tourism Research*, 22 (2): 313–27.

Creighton, M.R. (1995) 'Japanese craft tourism; liberating the crane wife', *Annals of Tourism Research*, 22 (2): 463–78.

Crompton, R. and Sanderson, K. (1990) *Gendered Jobs and Social Change*, London: Unwin Hyman.

Delphy, C. (1977) *The Main Enemy*, London: WRRC (Women's Research and Resources Centre).

Fairbairn-Dunlop, P. (1994) 'Gender, culture and tourism development in Western Samoa', in V. Kinnaird and D. Hall (eds) *Tourism: A Gender Analysis*, Chichester: Wiley.

García-Ramón, M.D., Canoves, G. and Valdovinos, N. (1995) 'Farm tourism, gender and the environment in Spain', *Annals of Tourism Research*, 22 (2): 267–82.

Graburn, N. (1983) 'Tourism and prostitution', *Annals of Tourism Research*, 10 (3): 437–42.

Hall, C.M. (1992) 'Sex tourism in South-East Asia', in D. Harrison (ed.) *Tourism and the Less Developed Countries*, London: Belhaven.

Hall, C.M. (1994) 'Gender and economic interests in tourism prostitution', in V. Kinnaird and D. Hall (eds) *Tourism: A Gender Analysis*, Chichester: Wiley.

Harrison, D. (1992) 'Tradition, modernity and tourism in Swaziland', in D. Harrison (ed.) *Tourism and the Less Developed Countries*, London: Belhaven.

Hartmann, H. (1979) 'Capitalism, patriarchy and job segregation by sex', in Z.R. Eisenstein (ed.) *Capitalist Patriarchy and the Case for Socialist Feminism*, New York: Monthly Review Press.

Hartmann, H. (1981) 'The unhappy marriage of Marxism and feminism: towards a more progressive union', in L. Sargent (ed.) *The Unhappy Marriage of Marxism and Feminism: A Debate on Class and Patriarchy*, London: Pluto.

Hennessy, S. (1994) 'Female employment in tourism development in South-West England', in V. Kinnaird and D. Hall (eds) *Tourism: A Gender Analysis*, Chichester: Wiley.

Himmelweit, S. and Mohun, S. (1977) 'Domestic labour and capital', *Cambridge Journal of Economics*, 1 (1): 15–31.

Kinnaird, V. and Hall, D. (1994) *Tourism: A Gender Analysis*, Chichester: Wiley.

Lee, W. (1991) 'Prostitution and tourism in South-East Asia', in N. Redclift and M.T. Sinclair (eds) *Working Women. International Perspectives on Labour and Gender Ideology*, London and New York: Routledge.

Leheny, D. (1995) 'A political economy of Asian sex tourism', *Annals of Tourism Research*, 22 (2): 367–84.

Leontidou, L. (1994) 'Gender dimensions of tourism in Greece: employ-ment, sub-cultures and restructuring', in V. Kinnaird and D. Hall (eds) *Tourism: A Gender Analysis*, Chichester: Wiley.

Meisch, L.A. (1995) 'Gringas and Otavaleños: changing tourist relations', *Annals of Tourism Research*, 22 (2): 441–62.

Mies, M. (1986) *Patriarchy and Accumulation on a World Scale*, London: Zed.

Momsen, J. Henshall (1994) 'Tourism, gender and development in the Caribbean', in V. Kinnaird and D. Hall (eds) *Tourism: A Gender Analysis*, Chichester: Wiley.

Moore, R.S. (1995) 'Gender and alcohol use in a Greek tourist town', *Annals of Tourism Research*, 22 (2): 300–13.

Morris, J. (1986) *Women Workers and the Sweated Trades: The Origins of Minimum Wage Legislation*, Aldershot: Gower.

Pateman, C. (1988) *The Sexual Contract*, Cambridge: Polity Press.

Picard, M. (1993) 'Cultural tourism in Bali: national integration and regional differentiation', in M. Hitchcock, V.T. King and M.G. Parnwell (eds) *Tourism in South-East Asia*, London and New York: Routledge.

Pruitt, D. and LaFont, S. (1995) 'For love and money: romance tourism in Jamaica', *Annals of Tourism Research*, 22 (2): 422–40.

Raymond, J. (1986) *A Passion for Friends: Toward a Philosophy of Female Affection*, London: Women's Press.

Rees, T. (1992) *Women and the Labour Market*, London and New York: Routledge.

Rich, A. (1983) 'Compulsory heterosexuality and lesbian existence', in A. Snitow, C. Stansell and S. Thompson (eds) *Powers of Desire: The Politics of Sexuality*, New York: Monthly Review Press.

Rubery, J. (1978) 'Structured labour markets, worker organization and low pay', *Cambridge Journal of Economics*, 2 (1): 17–36.

Sanfey, P. (1995) 'Insiders and outsiders in union models', *Journal of Economic Surveys*, 9 (3): 255–84.

Sinclair, M.T. (1991) 'Women, work and skill: economic theories and feminist perspectives', in N. Redclift and M.T. Sinclair (eds) *Working Women. International Perspectives on Labour and Gender Ideology*, London and New York: Routledge.

Sturdevant, S. Pollock and Stoltzfus, B. (1992) *Let the Good Times Roll. Prostitution and the U.S. Military in Asia*, New York: The New Press.

Swain, M. Byrne (1993) 'Women producers of ethnic arts', *Annals of Tourism Research*, 20 (1): 32–52.

Swain, M. Byrne (ed.) (1995) *Gender in Tourism*, Special issue of *Annals of Tourism Research*, 22 (2).

Swain, M. Byrne (1995) 'Gender in tourism', *Annals of Tourism Research*, 22 (2): 247–66.

Truong, T-D. (1990) *Sex, Money and Morality: Prostitution and Tourism in South-East Asia*, London and New Jersey: Zed.

Urry, J. (1990) *The Tourist Gaze: Leisure and Travel in Contemporary Societies*, London: Sage.

Walby, S. (1986) *Patriarchy at Work: Patriarchal and Capitalist Relations in Employment*, Cambridge: Polity Press.
Walby, S. (1988) 'Segregation in employment in social and economic theory' in S. Walby (ed.) *Gender Segregation at Work*, Milton Keynes and Philadelphia: Open University Press.
Walby, S. (1990) *Theorizing Patriarchy*, Oxford: Basil Blackwell.
Wilkinson, P.F. and Pratiwi, W. (1995) 'Gender and tourism in an Indonesian village', *Annals of Tourism Research*, 22 (2): 283–99.

Chapter 2

Gender takes a holiday
Representation in holiday brochures

Margaret Marshment

[Woman's] function after all is to sell a product. . . . She herself
is objectified. She becomes part of the packaging of the product –
or even the product itself.

(Dickey and Stratford, 1987: 75)

The objectification of women in advertising has long been the focus
of feminist critiques of media representation. Capitalism's use of the
sexualized female body to sell its products has been seen as
constituting a significant contribution to the reproduction of ideologies of sexism and hence of patriarchal relations.[1] Particular
criticism – and derision – was directed at those advertisements
employing the staple image of the 'pin-up' to sell products such
as cars and machine tools to men (Sharpe, 1976: 109). Since the
'pin-up', like the 'bathing beauty', conventionally consists of a
young, shapely woman in a swimsuit, it would not be surprising
to find this image featuring widely in publicity for holidays. Given
that a 'holiday', in British culture, usually connotes a beach holiday,
and that a swimsuit is what is worn on the beach, the image would
be motivated by this logic.

It does not appear, however, that the 'sexual sell' as such is
dominant in contemporary holiday publicity. There is no shortage
of images of women in this material, nor of swimsuits, but the
regimes of representation within which they appear are structured
to produce a range of meanings around gender and holidays that are
not necessarily sexual, nor which articulate the sexuality of women
to other discourses.

The 'holiday' is by now an established component of British
popular culture. Holiday tourism is big business, with a mass
market product, the package holiday, and a range of alternative

products aimed at niche markets. In the mass media, holidays constitute a significant and regular area of representation. Newspapers and magazines carry regular holiday/travel features, television and radio have weekly holiday/travel programmes (second only to soap operas in popularity, it is claimed), women's magazines do features on holidays as well as on beach fashion and beauty tips in their summer issues, and there are periodicals devoted entirely to holidays, such as the BBC's monthly *Holiday*. Advertising, except for small ads, tends to be concentrated in the post-Christmas period, although holiday iconography finds its way into advertising for other products, such as sun-tan creams or Bacardi rum. And then, of course, there are the scores of holiday brochures produced by the tour operators of package holidays which line the walls of travel agents in every high street.

PACKAGE HOLIDAYS

It is these brochures (covering the period 1993–1995) that are the focus of this analysis of the interface between constructions of 'the holiday' and constructions of gender. Available free, they are presumably read by choice, so we may assume a wide distribution to an interested readership, although that interest may be focused more on prices and dates than on the relatively incidental publicity material they also contain. The brochures are primarily concerned with providing this kind of detailed information to enable people already familiar with the structure of a 'package' holiday to select their precise destination and time of stay. It is the publicity material, however, which is visually dominant and most important in the construction of meanings.

The holiday market in general is most obviously distinguished along lines of class, either in terms of cost or in terms of 'taste' (see Bourdieu, 1984, Part III). This distinction is clearly visible in the differences between advertisements and features in respectively the 'quality' and tabloid press, or glossy women's magazines and the cheaper ones. Here, the former emphasize the distinctive holiday experiences available for those with money and/or the cultural capital to pursue luxury, authenticity or special interests (such as sailing or opera),[2] while the latter tend to stress the familiar pleasures of sand, sea and sun to be anticipated from a beach holiday. The package holiday is generally perceived to be a standardized product aimed at the mass market rather than a 'discriminating' public. The brochures largely confirm this, in that they offer predominantly beach holidays in Mediterranean resorts, with prices more dependent on the season than on the particular hotel or holiday. They do, however, also offer long-haul holidays, which are both more expensive and less exclusively beach-orientated, and one form of activity holiday (skiing), so that there is some reflection here of the general class/taste distinctions evident elsewhere.

The brochures fall into genres, distinguished by destination, type of holiday or type of holidaymaker. Thus, on the one hand, there are brochures devoted to the Mediterranean or particular Mediterranean countries, and on the other to 'long haul' holidays in more distant places; there are brochures devoted to skiing holidays, 'winter sun' holidays, 'city breaks' and cruises; and there are holidays aimed at the over 55s, at honeymooners and at the 18–30 age group. There are no holidays designed specifically for women. As John Urry observes, the 'holiday', unlike leisure, has been constructed in our culture as primarily based around 'the couple' (Urry, 1990: 140–144). Unlike markets for so many other goods and services (clothes, cosmetics, magazines and so on), the holiday market is not constructed along gender lines. This has the plus of constructing holidays as not gender-specific and thereby not excluding women as participants and consumers but, simultaneously, the minus of rendering invisible the economic and social differences between women and men that affect their ability to take holidays on the same basis. Even holiday features in women's magazines make no reference to women's particular interests or problems in taking holidays, and could equally well appear in the mainstream press. For 1996 Airtours announced a brochure cover featuring a single smiling woman, designed to resemble a woman's magazine cover and appeal to women as the major decision-makers in purchasing a holiday (*Financial Times*, 30.8.95). This is a major departure in terms of sales pitch, but the holiday product would appear to remain ungendered.

The overall design of the brochures is fairly uniform with a strongly visual front cover, a few pages of general publicity material at the beginning, and information on booking, flights, visas and vaccinations at the end. The bulk of the brochure is devoted to describing the available accommodation in various resorts, listing facilities and prices in small print surrounded by an assortment of small colour photographs which take up, on average, between a half and two-thirds of each page. Differences in style correlate more with the genre of the brochure than the tour operator.

THE WOMAN IN A SWIMSUIT

The front covers obviously constitute the most immediate invitation to potential holidaymakers. These all feature colour photographs, either a single full-page one, or a collage of smaller ones. Those that refer to the beach holiday usually feature, as might be expected, a beach, either as a general scene or as the setting for a family group or for one or two adults. The first of these is fairly straightforwardly iconic of what a beach holiday purports to offer – sand, sea and sun; the others employ representations of people to suggest the pleasures of this kind of holiday, through showing presumed holidaymakers with whom readers are invited to identify. They appear to use professional models to represent these holidaymakers, in as much as the people shown represent cultural ideals of male and female beauty – slim, tanned and usually blonde young women; muscular, tanned and usually blonde young men.

With the exception of brochures aimed at the older age group (which show a middle-aged couple, usually fully-clothed and often on a veranda),[3] the women on these covers, whether in a family group, in a couple or alone, is almost always wearing a swimsuit.[4] Here we may see the articulation of the 'pin-up' to specific discourses in the construction of holidays. First, there is the domestication of her sexuality within the family. 'Family' covers show a young couple with their (one, two or three) children, physically close to each other and laughing. The 'woman in a swimsuit' contributes to this definition of the ideal nuclear family as young, white, beautiful and happy. Her sexuality is not denied so much as made wholesome in the service of family fun. At the same time it is necessary to the glamorization of the family holiday in order to connote the luxury associated with a foreign holiday in the sun: a plump woman in glasses would not perform the same function any more than would a balding husband or crying children. It is not just, or even especially, the image of the woman that defines the family in this way, but it is this particular image of woman that contributes to this particular definition.

The other way in which the 'woman in a swimsuit' functions on the brochure covers occurs when she appears alone or in a couple. These covers tend to convey a more 'arty', up-market impression:

with fewer primary colours and less fussy print, they aim for a more elegant aesthetic. Unlike 'families', couples and women alone less often face the camera or laugh; rather, they gaze at each other or out to sea; they may be seen from the back or silhouetted against the sunset; the woman alone may also be reclining on the beach.[5] The holiday pleasures signified by these covers are those of relaxing in a warm climate in beautiful surroundings, linked to romance perhaps, but above all connoting the hedonism of idleness – especially when the woman is relaxing alone. It is notable, in fact, that while the woman can signify this pleasure when alone, the man can only do so in the company of a woman. It would seem that in our culture the conventional associations between beauty, pleasure, sexuality and femininity allow images of women to evoke these qualities in ways that images of men cannot. Despite tendencies towards the sexual aestheticization of men in certain genres of representation (see, for example, Moore, 1988), it seems that these images are not sufficiently established to signify, by themselves, qualities such as beauty, pleasure and sexuality in other contexts.

As a result, it is the 'woman in a swimsuit' that functions as a signifier of the beach holiday. Along with its other signifiers – the beach itself, the blue sky, the blue water of sea or pool, a palm tree perhaps – the woman in a swimsuit signifies the pleasures of idleness and luxury that certain representations of the beach holiday offer. There are no comparable images of men. Logically there is no reason why a handsome man lounging nearly naked on a beautiful beach cannot signify the same luxurious idleness. In our culture, however, it seems that only women can, on their own, embody this promise of pleasure. Not quite in the manner of the 'sexual sell': it is not she who is on offer, but what she represents; she is not part of the holiday package, but a signifier of it. Clearly, while this does not transform woman's sexuality into a product, it is only because of the strong conventional associations between femininity and aesthetic and sexual pleasure that this image of woman can signify pleasure in general in the context of holidays. In addition, a particular image of woman is required to perform this signifying role: she must conform to cultural definitions of beauty – young, slim and shapely – in order to embody the aestheticization of the holiday; and she must be white, if only to signify the attainment of that product of the holiday, a suntan. The sexual availability and passivity of the images are not lost, but rather articulated to a generalized sense of narcissistic self-indulgence. All these conventional connotations are therefore reproduced in the service of a more generalized promotion of a promise of pleasure.

THE 'SEXUAL SELL'

Where the 'sexual sell' is more clearly in evidence, it is inflected away from a direct address in terms of sexual availability. The brochure covers featuring an eroticized image of woman use, not photographs, but stylized drawings, with the implication that these are not images to be taken entirely seriously.[6] They do not quite qualify as postmodern irony, but, in eschewing realistic photographs, they refer perhaps self-consciously to cartoon pin-ups rather than soft pornography.

In the brochures for holidays aimed at the younger age group, such as Twentys or The Club, we do find more conventionally eroticized photographic images of women. Here the holidaymakers are visually far more dominant than the hotels or the resorts, suggesting that the social side of holidays is more important to this age group, an implication reinforced by the texts' emphasis on nightlife. All those represented are young, conforming to contemporary definitions of sexual attractiveness, in styles which owe much to teenage magazines concerned with fashion and/or pop music. Importantly, the young men represented are also coded for erotic appeal, with plenty of bare muscular torsos and moody looks, so that, while there are more images of young women in bikinis or mini skirts, displaying cleavages and long smooth legs, this sexualization of young women is not obviously addressed only to male viewers, but forms part of a coding of a lifestyle intended to appear fashionable, free and exciting. This is the only genre of brochure to show black people among the holidaymakers, although an average of one per brochure massively under-represents the proportion of young black people in the population.

It may be interesting to compare these particular brochures with examples from other media. Even in the tabloid newspapers, notorious for their exploitation of female sexuality, the context may often work against a reading simply in terms of a 'sexual sell'. For example, a *Daily Mirror* publicity feature for a holiday competition to 'Win Your Dream Holiday' (1.1.94) shows a back view of a young woman lying on a white beach at the sea's edge, tanned, wearing a red swimsuit and with wet hair. This could be read as offering a male reader the woman as his prize, identical with the holiday. But this is far from being the only, or perhaps the dominant, reading. It is not clear that this feature addresses a male spectator. The feature immediately above advertises the 'Weightwatchers New Diet' and shows a similarly shapely young woman in a swimsuit/ leotard. Here we assume that women readers are being addressed, in their desire to 'stay slim for ever!'. So perhaps women readers are also being invited to imagine themselves as the woman on the beach enjoying her 'dream holiday'. This reading is encouraged by the fact that this woman has the 'figure' of the fashion model found in women's magazines rather than the 'body' of the woman of pornography aimed at men.

A Virgin Holidays advertisement provides a different, and less typical, example. Here the bottoms of two young women are shown, hardly covered by their swimsuits, with the caption, 'Barefaced Chic'. The pun is porno-style, but its context in, for example, the *Holiday Destinations* magazine, allows it to be read as self-consciously so, and because pornography itself is not, these days, anything like as coy, encourages an ironic reading, and, in a climate of assumed sexual liberalism, one that is not necessarily addressed only to men. This jokey reference to sexual licence, addressed to both genders, is also the theme of the controversial 1995 Club Med advertising campaign.

In the context of holiday publicity, what these examples might suggest is that the 'sexual sell' needs, now, to be circumscribed by ambiguity or irony; that if twenty-five years of feminism have not destroyed sexism, in some mainstream contexts they have compelled it to adopt what are perhaps defensive strategies.

SUN AND SAFETY

On the inside pages of brochures for Mediterranean beach holidays the emphasis is overwhelmingly on the hotels. The exterior of almost every hotel listed is shown: usually white high-rise buildings with balconies, set against a matt blue sky with a foreground of blue sea or, more usually, the hotel swimming pool. Interiors feature bars, restaurants and bedrooms, while the hotel grounds show terrace cafés or, again, the pool. Photographs of the surrounding landscape or resort are relatively rare and consist mostly of beach scenes, with perhaps a scattering of iconic representations of place, such as a monument or a local market. The brief descriptions introducing particular countries or resorts tend to be very general and to emphasize weather and landscape, especially beaches, or tourist activities such as sports and nightlife; even where excursions are listed, these are seldom accompanied by photographs to entice the visitor to take them, while some brochures make almost no reference to a world outside the hotel compound. The emphasis is therefore very much on the 'holiday' rather than tourism.

There are plentiful photographs of the holidaymakers themselves within these compounds: apparently not professional models, but rather actual hotel guests. Although the number of poolside scenes mean that the majority are shown in swimwear, there is very little sense of eroticization of the image. If most are youngish and slimmish, they are not glamourized, not always even tanned, and plumper and/or older people are not excluded. Most do not look at the camera, or do so in the self-conscious manner found in holiday snaps. The invitation is not to gaze at them as ideal bodies representing a promise of beauty, glamour or sexual pleasure, but to identify with their experience of leisure. Potential customers are presumably expected to see these holidaymakers as ordinary British people like themselves, and – for the price of the package – to anticipate being in the same situation. As Cohen suggests, these are images designed to 'vicariously substitute for the observer of the image' (Cohen, 1993: 49).

Almost all are shown lounging around: rarely are they participating in any active pursuit: the pool is more for lying on or around than for swimming, and the sea is more for looking at. There is an occasional shot of a golf course or a couple walking on the beach, but mostly holidaymakers are shown sunbathing or drinking on the terrace or, yet again, by the pool. The passivity so often embodied in the image of the 'woman in a swimsuit' finds its analogue in the absence of activity in portrayals of the holiday-makers. Contrary to Linder's concept of the 'harried leisure class' (Linder, 1970), therefore, a holiday is here constructed as an opportunity to do nothing.

Nor is it constructed as an opportunity to meet people. Surprisingly perhaps, given the travel and accommodation structures of package holidays, the brochures do not suggest new social contacts as one of their attractions, which implies that the groups and couples depicted in them are holidaying together on the basis of a previously established relationship. And, just as they are seldom shown experiencing the landscape or culture of the holiday destination, so they are never shown socializing with local people.

Clearly, the tour operators are not targeting potential Shirley Valentines in their publicity. Far from offering the challenge of new experiences as an alternative to the routines of everyday life, these holidays offer the security of familiar companions in familiar surroundings. If traditional wisdom has it that what the British seek in Mediterranean holidays are the 'three S's' of sun, sea and sangria, it would seem that the tour operators have redefined these as sun, sloth and safety. With the 'pull' factors thus reduced, the 'push' factors would seem to be similarly reduced to an escape from work and the British weather. In their critique of the function of mass culture in capitalist society, Adorno and Horkheimer claim that the entertainment industry does not offer people an escape from the routines of work so much as a repetition of these routines in their leisure time: 'amusement under late capitalism is the prolongation of work' (Adorno and Horkheimer, 1977: 361). In as much as the hotel environment is offered as the dominant holiday experience, it would seem that these particular package holidays are similarly based on a difference from everyday life that is itself characterized by similarity to it.

DEFINING BRITISHNESS

In so far as the people photographed in the brochures are to be understood as representing 'ordinary' British holidaymakers, in that they are not unusually beautiful or glamorous, this constitutes a definition of 'ordinary' that is very restricted in terms of differences among the British population. There is an even distribution of females and males, and a fairly wide age range, from toddlers to late middle-age, but with a concentration around the thirties, and with noticeably few old people, babies or teenagers. There are other, perhaps more significant omissions: there are no disabled people, no pregnant women, no really fat people, and, above all, no black people. Ethnically these holidaymakers appear to be unambigu-ously 'Anglo-Saxon', frequently blonde and with no suggestion of the ethnic or cultural diversity of British society; not only are there no representatives of Britain's black or Asian communities, nor are there any who might be readily identified as from, say, Cypriot, Italian or Jewish communities. Of course, not all ethnic identities are visible in the person, and it may be that individuals photo-graphed here do originate from these communities. The point is that they do not signify this diversity. It is impossible to know how accurate this is as a reflection of those actually taking such holidays, but it is certain that these brochures' construction of 'a holiday' is in line with how certain ideologies of the British are constructed. That is, as white, able-bodied and heterosexual, and as clearly distinguishable from the 'foreigners' who people their holiday destinations.

There is no specific gender address in the brochures. The frequent use of the pronouns 'you' and 'your' could be singular or plural; there are no references to 'wives' or 'husbands', and the only references to family relationships concern those between parents and young children. These forms of address imply neither a gendered reader, nor (except in the case of families) a particular relationship between those holidaying together. But the actual organization and pricing of hotel accommodation, according to which the standard cost of a hotel room is based on double occupation, powerfully reinforces the general cultural expectation that people live in heterosexual couples and that they also holiday in heterosexual couples.[7] This implication is made explicit in the 'couple only' holidays, mostly located, it seems, in Caribbean resorts, which specify that the couple must consist of a man and a woman.[8]

These are the only holidays consistently to show hotel bedrooms with a double bed, with its suggestion of sexual intimacy, rather than twin beds. While in general the majority of bedrooms shown are occupied by a woman and a man, with or (more usually) without children, there is a significant sprinkling of photographs showing only one occupant, or showing two men or two women together. This pattern is repeated in the representation of holidaymakers in other hotel contexts, where the majority are shown in heterosexual pairings, families or gender-balanced groups. Again, some do show women or men either alone, with a companion of the same sex, or in groups of various combinations.

However dominant heterosexual coupledom may be, other relationships are not, therefore, explicitly excluded, and just what they might consist of is, in a sense, left open. Photographs without captions are inherently polysemic, so that two men shown sharing a drink might be read as husbands whose wives are elsewhere or as a gay couple. And the occasional image is rather more ambiguous: two women in bikinis smiling affectionately at each other by the pool, two men in shorts and t-shirts doing the same in the bar, are by no means explicitly gay images, though they might be seen as open to gay appropriation.

However, appropriation is a strategy of resistance; it assumes a norm that excludes, or is even hostile to, those doing the appropriating. It is not just the brochures that construct this norm, but the social context in which they are read. Contemporary British society, with its promotion of 'family values' (however unsuccessful in practice), would militate against readings that run counter to this heterosexual norm, unless the text invited us to do so. And while the brochures do not absolutely exclude such readings, neither do they invite them, so that their preferred meanings are such as to reinforce the society's ideological constructions of 'normal' relationships, and to do so within a broader construction of 'ordinary' British people in terms of able-bodiedness, age and ethnic identity.

SERVICE WITH A SMILE

In addition to representations of holidaymakers, the other people represented fall into two main, and sometimes overlapping, categories: those servicing the holidaymakers and those local inhabitants who are presented as part of the holiday experience. The former appear to be British when they occupy the role of the tour operator's representatives. Such images are fairly infrequent, are more usually women than men, are young, smiling to camera, and, with very few exceptions, white.

Locals occupying service roles are overwhelmingly waiters (serving drinks more often than food), followed by shopkeepers or market stallholders selling traditional food or craft products such as carpets and pottery. Finally, there are the entertainers, such as musicians or dancers. Only as dancers, in 'traditional' costume, are women more common than men. In all cases, the people function as part of the signification of a culture constructed as 'traditional'. But again, there are relatively few such images, especially in brochures dealing with Mediterranean holidays.

THE EXOTIC HOLIDAY

It is only in brochures advertising more distant destinations that the location of the holiday assumes an importance over the accommodation. Even here, some of the more cheaply produced ones, many devoted to the Caribbean, follow the 'beach holiday' format, though with rather more stress on palm-fringed beaches than hotel pools. Most, however, make considerably more reference to the country of destination, with fewer photographs of hotels and holidaymakers, and more of what are assumed to be the attractions of the location. The selling point of these 'long haul' holidays is not only the luxury of relaxing on tropical beaches, but also the difference represented by the 'exotic' geography and/or culture of their settings. The covers make this clear, with titles such as 'Distant Dreams' or 'Faraway Shores', offers of 'weddings in paradise' and claims to be 'more exotic, less expensive'.[9]

And it is here that the third category of representations of people are mostly to be found. Both inside the brochures and on the covers, the countries to be visited are offered up to the tourist gaze through a collage of photographs of monuments and artefacts, landscapes, animals and local inhabitants. The people, then, merge with, and form part of, the geographical and cultural landscape that constitutes the holiday experience. Most of these brochures cover a range of countries, each of which is signified by instantly recognizable images: the Great Wall for China, the Taj Mahal for India, the Pyramids for Egypt, and so on, together with others that have had less currency in our culture, such as the Sukhotai temple in Thailand or the Terracotta Army in China, but which, with repetition in the brochures, may well become equally familiar. These iconic monuments, as with those less frequently used ones in the Mediterranean brochures, are always associated with the past, preferably the distant past. On the other hand Hong Kong and Singapore, together with the USA and Australia, are characterized through images of cities which are not only modern, but ultra-modern, which itself signifies a form of the exotic, and which includes people only as an urban mass. Otherwise, exoticism is signified by an absence of the modern: everything from trains, tarmac and telegraph poles to jeans, t-shirts and transistor radios are excluded from representations of countries such as Mexico, Bali, Egypt, Thailand, Jamaica and so on. Even places such as Tiananmen Square, which might call to mind more recent historical events, with their political implications, are excluded. It is tradition, not history, that the signs of the past are intended to evoke. Unlike history, tradition is perceived as unchanging; as an intrinsic, almost natural, quality of a people.

Geographical distance clearly connotes cultural distance, and together they signify exoticism. The 'other' of the exotic is identified with nature rather than culture, with tradition rather than history, the past rather than the modern. This defines the 'other' in opposition to the assumed modern identity of the western tourist. Yet because the tourist is a holidaymaker rather than a traveller, this must be coded as simultaneously comfortable and safe, so that the 'other' is tamed through its contiguity with images that are both familiar and benign. This is achieved not only through photographs of modern luxury hotels and idyllic beaches, but through the regimes of representation employed in the depiction of the local people.

In order to facilitate instant recognition of the place signified, many of these images of people, like those of the monuments and natural features, amount to familiar stereotypes. Not, of course, by intention, derogatory stereotypes. On the contrary, they are designed to present the people and the countries they represent in a 'positive' light, as representing a difference that is sufficiently interesting and attractive to western tourists for them to pay to see them, but which is also by definition familiar.

Such representations fall into two main groups. The first covers people dressed in some form of 'national' costume signifying the particular country. These may be examples of ways of dressing in general use, such as Indian women's wearing of saris, which feature widely in representations of India, or they may be more confined to formal and/or festive occasions, such as the costumes worn by Thai or Hawaiian dancers, also frequently represented. The second group concerns images of people in work situations: here it is not the dress, but the occupation that signifies the local culture. Examples would include tea pickers or stilt fishermen in Sri Lanka and young buddhist monks in Thailand; all frequently used. In addition, there are representations of local people engaged in less country-specific craft occupations, such as pottery, fishing or agriculture, and in tourist-related occupations such as beach traders or entertainers. If politics and history are absent from representations of the country, the poverty of the people is transformed into the picturesque. Thus, a peasant woman toiling in the fields is captioned 'scenic Crete', while women picking tea or collecting firewood are included as examples of 'local colour'. And just as all signs of modernity are excluded from the images of their countries, so too are the people identified inside modernity, we do not see people working in factories, offices or department stores.

Representations of 'local' people, unlike those of holidaymakers who are shown mostly in couples or mixed-gender groups, always –

except for the occasional crowd scene – show them either alone or in same-gender groups. The waiter, shopkeeper or dancer, for example, is shown in her/his function in relation to the tourist as a lone worker; while groups of monks, fishermen or marketwomen, for example, are displayed as evidence of the local culture. What this fails to suggest, therefore, is the existence in the host culture of a home life, or of familial or sexual relations. It is not only that this host culture is offered up in segments to the tourist gaze, but that these segments omit those social relations of family, romance and sexuality that the publicity itself foregrounds in its representations of the tourists. It is not only technology, therefore, that defines the modernity of the tourist, but social relations themselves; in particular, the nuclear family and heterosexual romance, but generally any relations internal to the host society, including those of consumerism. While the tourist/holidaymaker is automatically portrayed as a consumer/voyeur of other environments and culture, the members of the host society are shown only as workers and/or objects of the tourist gaze. As a result, any social relations imputed to the host society (such as those involved in religion or carnival) are portrayed as 'other' than the essentially modern relations enjoyed by the tourist. None of these meanings are addressed to a gendered spectator. Nor are there obvious distinctions to be made between the way in which representations of men and women are employed in communicating them. With one exception, there is a more or less even spread of representation of men, women and children in images of local people in the brochures. What is important is that where gender relations are foregrounded in representations of the tourists, they are all but eliminated in those of the host culture. Even so, the exception mentioned above points to one subtle difference which suggests that gender has one specific function in the construction of the 'other'.

A GENDERED AESTHETIC

The Tradewinds 1995 brochure is the only one to feature considerably more representations of women than men (in a ratio of more than 2:1). This brochure is a high quality product, with crisp elegant layout and high-definition photographs, clearly aiming to signify the quality of its holidays through the aesthetic quality of its publicity. It devotes little space to pictures of holidaymakers, hotels or pools – on many pages, none at all. The focus instead is on the tourist attractions of the holiday destinations: landscape, wildlife, architecture, artefacts and people. Most sections include at least one photograph of a local person smiling to camera. Some of these are photographs of men (an old Chinese man or a steel band musician), but the overwhelming majority are young women or girls. Often they wear some kind of 'national' costume, and are always beautiful. None, however, are overtly sexual images: they are mostly head-and-shoulder shots of demurely clothed women, with smiles that are reassuring rather than inviting. The potential sexuality of the image of a young woman is articulated to offer, not sex itself, but beauty, friendliness and difference.

The front cover is rather different, but may suggest how these images function in the context of holiday tourism. It consists of a full-page photograph of a young woman wearing 'traditional' oriental dress. This is an 'art'-style photograph: eschewing the primary colours of most travel brochures, it is in muted shades of gold, orange and straw; the focus is so soft as simultaneously to give the impression of a painting and to appear to veil the woman – presumably a suggestion of the stereotypical 'mystery of the east'. But she is not coded for erotic effect: only her head and shoulders are shown, and only her face and neck are visible; she is photographed in profile, gazing off the page and thus not engaging the look of the spectator. The 'mystery' of her demure femininity is being employed, not to offer an exotic sexuality to a male spectator, but rather to offer an aestheticized experience of 'the other' to an ungendered western spectator.

The aestheticized quality of this cover is exceptional, but it does point to a more general feature of the way in which photographs of people are used in these up-market brochures to connote a geographical and cultural 'otherness'. The fact that this particular image, and those of women inside the brochure, occur in a context of aestheticized pictures of landscape and animals, architecture and artefacts, suggests that their function is also importantly to represent the beautiful and to render the 'other' as a pleasurable, comfortable experience. In the context of ethnic 'otherness', native women do not signify anything radically different from what is signified by native men, because of the ways in which British culture has constructed both gender and race along parallel oppositions of the 'natural' and 'emotional' against the 'masculine' and 'white' norms of civilisation and reason. But the aesthetic, it seems, even in this context is still associated with femininity rather than masculinity. In addition, women from even the most exotically different cultures may be considered as embodying a less potential threat than might similarly 'exotic' men. The Tradewinds brochure contains two large photographs of this more threatening exotic, in the form of a Masai herdsman with spear and an extreme close-up of the painted face of a South Pacific man. The ideologies which associate women with physical beauty and docility are employed in taming the disturbing potential of the 'other' embodied in these images of 'primitive' manhood.

CONCLUSION

What this analysis suggests is that, while gender is not at first sight a dominant factor in the construction of the meanings of holidays in British culture, there are important ways in which it does, nevertheless, function in this context. The brochures do not address a gendered reader/potential consumer; nor is there a notable imbalance between male and female in their representations of people. However, it is important, first, in the construction of definitions of Britishness: the assumed heterosexuality of the couples represented, associated with the ideals of a companionate marriage and the nuclear family, contributes to the establishment of a norm of 'ordinariness' constructed across a range of other qualities – able-bodiedness, body size, attractiveness, age, class and, above all, ethnicity – which defines the 'ordinary' British holidaymaker, with which presumed 'ordinary' readers are invited to identify and which renders the holiday environment familiar, and therefore safe. That pleasure is associated culturally with women, rather than men, enables women's bodies – specifically, the image of the 'woman in a swimsuit' – to signify the particular pleasures of the beach holiday. And that beauty is associated with the female and not only facilitates this signification of pleasure, but also permits the use of representations of women 'of colour' to aestheticize and tame the 'other' as the object of the tourist gaze.

This, I would suggest, demonstrates how deeply embedded in our culture is the gendering of concepts. On the one hand, it is evident that the ideological structures which associate women with particular qualities to the exclusion of others (leisure rather than work, beauty rather than intelligence or strength) remain very powerful ones. So powerful that certain images of women can themselves connote these qualities. But only certain images: female beauty continues to be very narrowly defined. The 'woman in a swimsuit' can only signify the beach holiday as a desirable experience if she is young, slim and white; and the black woman can only tame the threat of the 'other' if she is young, slim and demure.

At the same time, it would seem that concepts such as pleasure and beauty are themselves impoverished through their conventional embodiment in a narrow range of images. Pleasure and beauty are sufficiently abstract qualities to permit of a myriad of associations, yet the pleasures connoted by the 'woman in a swimsuit' are as narrowly defined as she herself is. Similarly, ideas of difference and diversity are sadly diminished by a construction of the 'other' that is not only dehistoricized and depoliticized, but also contained as a spectacle for the aestheticized curiosity of the tourist. Of course, the discourses of holiday/tourism will have their boundaries, which might logically exclude certain dimensions of history, politics and culture, but the world of the brochures is constructed on such a narrow base, with so much repetition of images, and such a sense of cosy passivity, that its final effect is particularly claustrophobic.

CODA

This analysis has examined only British holiday brochures. However, a brief comparison with a similar range of holiday brochures from other Western European countries (Germany, France, Italy, Spain) suggests that an analysis of these would yield very similar results. There are some stylistic variations, but there is the same emphasis on hotels, pools, beaches and holidaymakers; a comparable use of the 'woman in a swimsuit'; and very considerable overlap in the images used to signify particular tourist destinations, including a similar use of representations of people.

It would seem, then, that the cultural construction of a 'holiday' is common to much of Western Europe. A significantly different construction is offered in the brochures produced by Japanese tour operators for a Japanese public. While these follow much the same general format, the predominant images are those of the tourist destination itself, with photographs of landscapes, cityscapes and tourist attractions, including works of art (such as paintings or stained glass windows) and cultural events (such as the Venice carnival). The emphasis is clearly on tourism rather than holiday. Indeed, the concept of a 'holiday' in the European sense of sun, sand and sea is absent from these brochures, for while there are some photographs of hotels (mostly interiors), there are almost none of pools or beaches.

There is a commensurate absence of representations of holiday-makers; and when they do occur they are almost always shown as white westerners, not Japanese. This is so even when the tourists depicted are clearly intended to represent potential customers, as in honeymoon holidays. This has the effect of erasing the distinction between tourists and locals in European/American contexts, although this distinction is maintained – and in exactly the same terms as in European brochures – in Asian, African and Caribbean contexts. Given that the word 'holiday' often appears in English in the brochures, it may be suggested that it signifies something that is perceived as a western phenomenon, identified with the modernity of western industrialized societies. If that is so, it is interesting that the only category of Japanese people to appear on the brochure covers are young women.

NOTES

1 See, for example, Sharpe, S., *Just Like a Girl: How Girls learn to be Women*, 1976, chapter 3, 'Reflections from the media'.
2 While there is considerable overlap between the 'tabloid' and the 'quality' press in the types of holidays advertised, the latter include more small ads in respect of, for instance, rented cottages and activity holidays such as cycling, walking, sailing or golf. There are also more advertisements for 'cultural' holidays, such as Nile cruises, (*Sunday Telegraph*, 2.1.1994) the Verona Opera (*Observer*, 2.1.1994) or the Venice Carnival (*Independent on Sunday*, 2.1.1994). Overall, these are not necessarily more expensive holidays, but like the features in the 'quality' press, lay rather more stress on 'authenticity' than on fun.
3 For example: Thomson, Young at Heart, October 1993–April 1994. More recent brochures also feature such couples in pools, though usually only head-and-shoulders shots – for example, Cosmos, Golden Times, November 1995–April 1996; Airtours, Golden Years, Winter 94–95.
4 For example: Aspro Holidays, Summer Sun, 1994; Cosmos, Summer Sun, March–October 1994; Unijet, Summer Sun, Summer 1994; and, a more up-market image without laughter, Airtours, Summer Sun, March–October 1994.
5 See for example: Olympic Holidays, Cyprus, Summer 1994; Airtours, Cyprus, Summer 1994; Enterprise, Tropical, Winter 1994/95.
6 The Airtours Caribbean brochures for 1994 and 1995 have stylized drawings of swimsuit-clad women on their covers.
7 This also works to discriminate against all groups, including families, consisting of odd numbers of people, with the implication, perhaps, that 'pairing off' is the dominant and desirable structure of all relationships.

8 Thomson's Worldwide brochure, November 1993–October 1994.
9 Cosmos, Thomson, Kuoni, respectively, 1994/95.

REFERENCES

Adorno, T. and Horkheimer, M. (eds) (1986) 'The culture industry: enlight-
enment as mass deception', in *The Dialectic of Enlightenment*, 2nd
edition, London: Verso.
Bourdieu, P. (1984) *Distinction: A Social Critique of the Judgement of
Taste*, London and New York: Routledge.
Cohen, E. (1993) 'The study of tourist images of native people: mitigating
the stereotype of the stereotype', in D.G. Pearce, and R.W. Butler (eds),
Tourism Research: Critiques and Challenges, London and New York:
Routledge.
Dickey, J. and Stratford, T. (eds) (1987) *Out of Focus*, London: The
Women's Press.
Linder, S.B. (1970) *The Harried Leisure Class*, New York and London:
Columbia University Press.
Moore, S. (1988) 'Here's looking at you kid', in L. Gamman and M.
Marshment (eds), *The Female Gaze*, London: The Women's Press.
Sharpe, S. (1976) *Just Like a Girl: How Girls Learn to be Women*,
Harmondsworth: Penguin.
Urry, J. (1990) *The Tourist Gaze: Leisure and Travel in Contemporary
Societies*, London: Sage.

Chapter 3

Women's employment in UK tourism
Gender roles and labour markets

Kate Purcell

WOMEN'S EMPLOYMENT IN TOURISM: THE BROAD PICTURE

In common with most of Western Europe, tourism-related employment in the UK is one of the few sectors of industry and commerce to have experienced an overall increase in job opportunities throughout the 1980s and early 1990s despite recessionary fluctuations (ETB/IMS 1986; NEDO 1992; HCTC 1994; European Commission 1994). This trend is projected to continue into the twenty-first century (Horwath and Horwath 1988, IER 1994). In the UK, the sector has been one of the fastest areas of employment growth (Metcalf 1987) and in the 1980s, three-quarters of this growth was represented by women's jobs — mainly part-time, insecure, low-status and low-paid personal service and clerical employment (HOST Consultancy 1991). Projections suggest, however, that tourism and leisure are also likely to be the only major growth area of full-time employment opportunities for women in the 1990s (Parsons 1992: 109).

The rate of employment growth in this complex, fragmented sector has varied among regions, ranging from 75 per cent in the South East of England to 32 per cent in the North (HOST Consultancy 1991: 17). Employment in the tourism sector is notoriously difficult to define comprehensively (Department of Employment 1987: 336). Industries which are primarily dependent upon tourism, such as hospitality and travel agencies, also provide services for non-tourism industries. On the other hand, consumer demand in production and service industries not directly concerned with tourism products fluctuates according to the fortunes of the tourism industry, particularly in localities which attract significant numbers of tourists and/or operate in economically peripheral areas (Medlik 1989). For example, research in Looe, Cornwall – a typical UK seaside resort – has found that business establishments in all sectors depended upon tourism to a greater or lesser extent (Hennessy *et al.* 1986: 25).

There is no single UK agency responsible for promoting tourism or monitoring tourism-related employment (NEDO 1992: 85). Government employment statistics are thus not classified in a way conducive to identification and aggregation of relevant occupations or analysis of trends, so no such analysis is routinely undertaken. Parsons (1992: 103) points out that there have been widespread inconsistencies among classifications used by different agencies and researchers, leading to conflicting analysis and interpretation, deriving from the fact that: 'The sector is essentially a composite of *consumer* rather than the more easily classified sectoral *economic* activity and is not easily differentiated in terms of standard industrial (or occupational) classifications'.

To add to the complexity, the sector is disproportionately characterized by 'informal economy' employment, particularly with regard to part-time and seasonal work of the kinds most often done by women. Hennessy (1994: 44), researching women's tourism-related employment in Cornwall, found extensive evasion of national insurance contributions, which suggests that recorded economic activity rates almost certainly underestimate tourism employment, particularly 'non-standard' employment disproportionately undertaken by women – casual employment, part-time and undeclared 'second jobs' and unregistered bed and breakfast businesses.

It is none the less worth looking at the most recent relevant statistics available, because they clearly indicate the extent to which the sector is gendered. The direct tourism employment sector has been most usefully defined (ETB/IMS 1986) as comprising three sectors of 'enabling activities' which facilitate tourism consumption: accommodation and catering; travel and passenger transport; and tourism, leisure and related activities. Figure 3.1 examines the ratios of males and females within these sectors and their main sub-sectors.

It can be seen from the disproportionate distributions of males and females within and among these sub-sectors of the tourism industry that accommodation and catering (generally speaking, the commercial sector of the hospitality industry, and the largest tourism-related

sector) is characterized by a numerically female-
force, nearly three-quarters of which is employ
hospitality sector as a whole has been claimed
largest sector of the British economy, estimat
million people in 1992 (HCTC 1994: 34). As
the sub-sectors where women predominate to the
also tend to be characterized by greater incidence of par
employment. Within this workforce, however, there is further
gender segmentation, as will be discussed in detail later in this
chapter.

Figure 3.1 The gendering of employment in tourism and leisure
(March 1995)

	% Male	% Female	% of females who are Part-time
Accommodation or catering activities (Total jobs = 1,077,600)			
Hotel trade and other tourist accommodation	40.00	60.00	(55.5)
Restaurants, cafés etc.	41.2	58.8	(69.8)
Public houses and bars	32.5	67.5	(83.1)
Night-clubs and licensed clubs	39.8	60.2	(85.6)
Total	**38.0**	**62.0**	**(72.4)**
Travel organizations and carriers (Total jobs = 844,500)			
Railways	87.6	12.4	(11.3)
Other inland transport	85.2	14.8	(39.8)
Sea transport and transport support services	77.2	22.8	(16.7)
Air transport	61.2	38.8	(14.5)
Miscellaneous transport and storage (not elsewhere specified)	54.1	45.9	(26.0)
Total	**75.7**	**24.3**	**(26.4)**
*Tourism, related leisure and associated services** (Total jobs = 193,000)			
Sport and other leisure services	51.6	48.4	(61.4)
Libraries, museums, art galleries etc.	29.2	70.8	(50.2)
Other community services	36.9	63.1	(61.5)
Total	**47.9**	**52.1**	**(58.9)**

Source: *Employment Gazette*, July 1995, S11, Table 1.4
Note: * Previous analyses have also included theatres, radio and television,
but this category is no longer identified in published tables.

onversely, the travel organizations and carriers sector is predominantly a male preserve, with men constituting three out of four employees in 1995, although women's share of the workforce increased somewhat in the 1980s (HOST Consultancy 1991: 30). Most women in this sector are employed full-time, in clerical jobs in travel agencies, as tour operators or transport administrators, or in personal service jobs in transport or resorts. There is, however, some indication of change in recent years. Women ranged from less than 8 per cent of railway employees in 1989 to two-thirds of airline cabin crew, whereas the comparable proportions in 1995 were 12 per cent and nearly 80 per cent. Privatization of air, rail and inland passenger transport in the late 1980s and early 1990s was justified on the basis of the pursuit of efficiency, flexibility and productivity, which has led to a decline in permanent full-time posts for both men and women and a small but significant increase in part-time employment in some of these occupations. Rubery and Fagan (1993: 95) suggest that recent increases in women's employment on the railways has been 'in part to change the culture to a more customer service-orientated approach, and possibly to change the employment system to a less regulated and institutionalised internal labour market prior to privatisation'. In fact, catering services were the first part of British Rail to be privatized.

Finally, tourism, related leisure and associated services accounts for the remainder of the enabling industries. Figure 3.1 reveals a more balanced gender distribution in this category than in the other two. Employment in this group is characterized by greater likelihood of professional or vocational qualification but as in all three sub-sectors, women are more likely than men to be found in relatively low-level personal service and clerical posts and, although increasingly entering the industry with professional or vocational qualifications, substantially less likely than men to be found at senior levels (White 1988, Bacon and Lewis 1990). Women are also most likely to be employed in libraries, museums, art galleries and heritage attractions mainly in occupations offering short-term seasonal work rather than long-term career prospects. Over half of all female employees in this sub-sector are employed part-time; a higher proportion in sport, other leisure services and other community services. Thus, as in the occupationally sex-segmented labour market as a whole, the tourism industry – particularly the accommodation and catering part of it – remains one of the most significant areas of female concentration.

In all of these 'enabling industries' women's role is thus predominantly in the low-paid, low status, clerical, interactive service and accommodation and catering service occupations – jobs rather than careers, where women compete with other disadvantaged workers in secondary rather than the primary labour markets. Employment structures and pressures leading to occupational segregation and role performance are highly complex and far from homogeneous (Metcalf 1987), with wide diversities among subsectors, between and within localities and even within fairly narrowly specified occupational groups.

ACCOMMODATION AND CATERING

For the purposes of this chapter, I propose to concentrate on employment in accommodation and catering, which are the dominant employment sectors within tourism (Baum 1993: 220) and the major enabling services provided by women in all the tourism subsectors. Bagguley (1991) analysed employment change in the UK hospitality industry between 1951 and 1981 to monitor gender ratios in different occupational groups and concluded that different explanations need to be found to explain successive phases of change, related to industrial, functional and hierarchical gender segregation. Between 1951 and 1971, women's employment in the industry fell as a result of technical innovation – mechanization of routine service work due to the widespread introduction of 'labour-saving' technology such as commercial dishwashers and waste disposal units (DE 1971: 25, Smith 1986: 35–7). In the 1970s, the occupational structure of the industry changed, rather, in response to deskilling of the cooking process, with the introduction of pre-prepared foods in commercial catering (Chivers 1973: 650–1): thus leading to less demand for 'craftsmen chefs and cooks' and a proportionate increase in the employment of women (Bagguley 1991: 615) with a narrower range of duties, less skill and lower earnings. Women have thus been increasingly recruited into jobs which are classified as unskilled (Rees and Fielder 1992, Rubery and Fagan 1993: 99).

Industry statistics chart the subsequent increased levels in employment and relative stability of gender segmentation (HCITB 1984, Guerrier 1986, HCTC 1984). Within the sector, women remain horizontally segregated into particular jobs and areas of operation, and vertically segregated into relatively low status and skilled occupations (HCITB 1987; Crompton and Sanderson 1989; HCTC 1994). Employment statistics for hotels and catering are regularly monitored by the Hotel and Catering Training Company (HCTC), formerly the Hotel and Catering Industry Training Board (HCITB). Hotel and catering employment includes institutional catering such as industrial, educational and health service catering services. As in the commercial sector, women employed in these areas are disproportionately found in the lowest occupational groups, but they are also more likely to be in professional or managerial posts than women in most other sectors (HCTC 1994). I will thus focus as far as possible on employment in the commercial sector, to attempt to obtain a picture of the structure and processes of women's employment in tourism-related hospitality which, for the most part, means hotels, restaurants, fast-food outlets, clubs and pubs; the provision of food and accommodation in travel, tourism and leisure services.

The most recent published statistics reveal that although women were 62 per cent of the total commercial sector workforce in 1992, their ratios in terms of occupational categories ranged from 39 per cent of publicans and 49 per cent of restaurant managers to 87 per cent of catering assistants, 80 per cent of kitchen porters and 74 per cent of travel attendants (HCTC 1994: 37). Part-time employees (working less than 30 hours per week) were in the majority – 55 per cent of the commercial sector overall – but were concentrated further within pubs and bars and clubs (over 80 per cent) and recreational/cultural outlets (approximately 70 per cent). The most striking aspect of part-time employment in hotels and catering is how *very* part-time it frequently is. Over a third of the industry's officially recorded employees worked fifteen hours or less per week in 1991 (Watson 1992: 546). Only in travel-related catering did full-time employees out number part-timers (ibid.: 40). This is particularly ironic given that the industry is reputedly one where the requirement to work long hours is often used as a reason why women do not make careers in it (Guerrier 1986). There would appear to be a particularly marked bifurcation between careers and jobs in the sector, with many supervisory and management jobs (for example, in fast food outlets and smaller catering establishments) at the 'job' rather than 'career' end of the spectrum in terms of reward, security and career development prospects, despite their managerial job-titles and responsibilities.

'WOMEN'S WORK', OR 'WORK FOR WOMEN'?

Given that the industry is essentially engaged in 'offering the amenities of the private or household sphere for sale in the public market' (Crompton and Sanderson 1989: 135), it is perhaps not surprising that women predominate in it. Caring for the comfort and welfare of others and preparing and serving food are quintes-sentially sex-typed 'women's work' calling for the exercise of tacit skills widely assumed to reflect 'inherent aptitudes' possessed by the majority of women (Walsh 1991: 112), developed in female gender socialization (Sharpe 1976) and household divisions of labour (Novarra 1980, Gershuny *et al.* 1994). 'Emotional labour' (Hochs-child 1983) – the implicit or explicit requirement within a job specification to control personal emotional responses and manage or manipulate the emotional well-being of customers or clients – is a significant aspect of many jobs in the industry. One of the char-acteristics of women's role in the overall human division of labour has been argued by classic sociological and psychological theorists to be an aptitude for 'affective' responsibilities. I propose to argue, however, that an analysis of women's employment in tourism-related hospitality reveals particularly clearly that there are three main elements determining or predisposing employers to recruit women for particular types of work: labour price, sex and gender. Thus, 'women's jobs' fall predominantly into one of three cate-gories: 'contingently gendered jobs' – which happen to be mainly done by women but for which the demand for labour is gender-neutral; 'sex-typed jobs', where sexuality or other attributes assumed to be sex-related (and certainly, are *gender*-related) are explicit or implicit parts of the job specification; and 'patriarchally prescribed jobs', where patriarchal practice determines and pre-scribes appropriate job incumbency. Many sectors in the industry have elements of more than one of these, but for analytic purposes it is instructive to consider the categories as ideal types which have a firm grounding in reality. The first is identical to Crompton and Sanderson's concept of 'crowded' jobs, but the second and third provide a more developed analysis than hitherto of the range of jobs where gender *is* an attribute demanded by employers, but on the basis of different criteria.

CONTINGENTLY GENDERED JOBS

As Crompton and Sanderson (1990: 155–8) have discussed, a significant proportion of the jobs where women predominate in the industry reflect their labour market position as disadvantaged rather than sex-typed workers. Their research findings suggest that gendered divisions of labour in the industry may be unstable, resting on employers' perceptions of economic advantage rather than gendered preferences: they want *cheap* workers, without being concerned, on the whole, whether these are male or female: though low-paid workers, particularly part-time employees, are most often women. Leidner (1993: 50–1), in considering the archetypical deskilled catering employees of recent years, McDonald's operative level staff, discussed how the company adjusted to a shortfall in its preferred labour supply:

> as the McDonald's chain has grown faster than the supply of teenagers, the company has also tried to attract senior citizens and housewives as workers. What people in these groups have in common is a preference or need for part-time work, and therefore a dearth of employment options. Because of this lack of good alternatives, and because they may have other means of support for themselves and their dependents, many people in these groups are willing to accept jobs that provide less than subsistence wages.

Thus, for such routine service jobs, at least, it is plausible to postulate that employers seek out the reserve army of labour which can be called upon during periods of relatively high demand and dispensed with, largely through natural wastage, when demand falls (Bruegel 1982; Beechey 1987).

In fact, the hospitality industry is notorious for high labour turnover at all levels (Wood 1992) and the extent to which this is a problem for the industry (Johnston 1985) or a useful facilitator of flexibility (Riley 1991) has been the subject of lively (and largely unresolved) debate, although the recession has clearly had the effect of slowing down frictional turnover (HCTC 1994: 8). Women have traditionally provided labour as required, conveniently leaving the active labour force at the end of the season and the female workforce has largely been relied upon to shrink by natural wastage when demand is relatively low. Increasing casualization of employment contracts throughout the 1980s has further enabled employers to use employees flexibly with no commitment to provide continuity when demand for services fluctuates (Rubery and Fagan 1993: 96).

Hennessey (1994) interviewed 125 women working in Looe during the 1984 tourism season, two-thirds of whom were found to be in seasonal employment. These women were mainly engaged in restaurants and cafés, shop work, cleaning and bar work, clearly providing a flexible and easily disposable workforce, but nearly two-thirds of the seasonal workers had worked for the same employer for over two seasons and a fifth for six or more years. Most of these jobs are likely to have been contingently gendered jobs, but their attraction of women is, in a high proportion of cases, based upon the women's capacity to survive between seasons as dependents of a breadwinner wage-earner, illustrating clearly how patriarchy and employers' economic rationality combine to reinforce both the public and the private gendered status quo.

Jobs predominantly undertaken by women have invariably been evaluated as involving little skill and accorded low status and reward, regardless of their inherent labour processes and whether or not they are intrinsically sex-typed in terms of job-content (Phillips and Taylor 1980). Gabriel (1988) has argued that work in the hospitality industry as a whole is stigmatized because of its associations with personal servitude; an image reinforced by its reliance upon a substantial peripheral workforce consisting, for the most part, of 'disadvantaged workers' – women (particularly part-time employees), ethnic minority employees, casual and transient workers, a significant proportion of whom have been alleged to be 'social misfits' who are attracted to hotel work in particular because of their lack of integration to normal family life and the community (Wood 1992: 18–22).

Contrary to this, Walsh (1989, 1991) has pointed out that most part-time, casual and temporary work in hospitality is done by women whose reliability and commitment belies the stereotype and whose work 'far from being peripheral to productivity, is central to it . . . purchased [efficiently by employers] on an 'as needed' or 'just in time' basis' (Walsh 1991: 113). Crompton and Sanderson (1990: 149–50) give the employment history of 'Valerie'; a banqueting waitress 'not . . . in any way exceptional' who had been a regular casual worker for the same employer for ten years, alternating between part-time and full-time employment, including split shift working. Such workers, of course, have considerably less employment rights than permanent employees, in an industry characterized by 'outdated' human resource management, which has been held largely responsible for the 'self-inflicted nature of many of the sector's recruitment and retention problems', where less than a quarter of employees have a written offer of employment or formal contract (Parsons 1992: 105; Price 1994).

Added to this, whether jobs are constructed by employers, or inadvertently 'end up as' female or male dominated as a result of labour supply factors, their resultant gender-segmented identity has the effect of attracting or repelling potential recruits, leading to self-replicating 'job-gendered' divisions of labour (Scott 1995: 239). Leidner (1993: 181) observes that work organizations are locations where 'the gender segregation of jobs helps sustain the notion that women and men have essentially different characters'.

In order to understand stability and change, however, the evolution of the employment in the industry needs to be considered within the labour market as a whole. Lovering (1994) explored the impact of economic restructuring within one locality (Swindon) on the gendering of employment, using case studies representing a range of industries, including commercial catering. He found that at 'Motormeals' – his motorway catering service area – 'The work was described by the manager as like much of the catering industry, "hot, sticky, mucky and low paid" and this is why it was performed mainly by women' Lovering 1994: 346). Thus depressingly reminiscent of Whyte's (1948: 33–5) findings in his classic study of the industry in post-war America. However, although a combination of occupational sex-typing by both employers and jobseekers, reinforced by the economic constraint of low pay, led to the perpetuation of gendered custom and practice, Lovering sees employers' increasing preoccupation with improving service as a potential challenge to it. Specialization and diversification within sectors is reflected in the *niche marketing* of 'specialist' products supposedly demanded by the increasingly sophisticated, affluent and demanding 'post-modernist' consumers (Urry 1990) who form the majority of the industry's customers; and provision of such a variety of products and services requires widening diversification of skills, knowledge and competence within each sector and often, within organizations.

The change in the nature and range of the hospitality product has involved a general move towards less seasonal demand, as conference and leisure business complement a more diverse range of tourism products. Lovering suggests that the net effect will be the introduction of new internal labour market opportunities based upon 'sex-neutral, meritocratic selection criteria' (Lovering 1994: 350), like the increasing importance of formal credentials (Crompton and Sanderson 1990, Purcell and Quinn 1995), which has allowed for at least the possibility of more equal job opportunities, if over a somewhat restricted range. However, the 'sex-neutral, meritocratic criteria' he cites, 'social skills, such as the ability to work in teams' and 'leadership qualities' (Lovering 1994: 347), could be argued to be neither sex-neutral nor meritocratic, given that they both rely on subjective and ideologically imbued criteria. Previous research findings in the hospitality and leisure industries (Guerrier 1986, Hicks 1990, Adkins 1995) suggest that such criteria are likely to reinforce rather than challenge sex-typed or patriarchally prescribed occupations.

SEX-TYPED OCCUPATIONS

The tourism industry has a history of paternalistic individualism where personal relationships and 'personality' have been more important in employment and industrial relations than formal quali- fications or collective agreements (Whyte 1949, CIR 1971, Wood 1992). A hotel manager interviewed by Hicks (1990: 356) claimed to hire management recruits 'only on personality' and this is perhaps a neat reinforcement of Filby's (1992) reflection that 'personality' very often is a codified shorthand for sexual attractiveness and/or gender-specific tacit skills and attributes. Of the leisure sector organization he studied, he was told by a male manager that recruitment of female staff was informed by 'a "height for weight" principle'. Filby was talking about informal job specifica- tions in another part of the leisure sector (betting shops), but if managers believe that men and women have very different attri- butes, orientations and potential, then what they mean by 'the right personality for the job' will almost certainly have implicit gendered sub-texts, whether they are looking for a bookmaker's clerk, a receptionist or a senior manager.

Adkins (1995: 109) reproduces the job specifications for employ- ees at 'Globe Hotel' where she discovered profoundly gendered explicitly different requirements for different jobs according to whether recruits were normally male or female. Thus, the specifica- tion for waitresses was '*attractive*, average weight and height, must have enthusiastic attitude', whereas for barmen, it was '*strong*, average weight and height, very smart, able to communicate well with general public, enthusiastic and helpful manner' (my emphasis). She observed that for all the 'female' interactive service jobs (including chambermaid) 'attractiveness' was a criterion of appointment and 'the specifications related to the gender of the occupants of the occupations, rather than to the requirements of the occupations themselves' (ibid.: 111).

Like others who have researched women's employment in the hospitality industry, Adkins found clear employer attempts to control the presentation of women employees in terms of clothing, make-up and prescribed behaviour (Spradley and Mann 1975; Hey 1986; Williams 1988; Leidner 1993). She observed (Adkins 1995: 119, 122) that men were more likely to be reprimanded in relation to behaviour and women in relation to appearance – largely in terms of failure to conform to the organizations' standards of 'normal' and 'attractive' presentation. Hochschild (1983: 96), similarly, reported that potential air stewardesses were required to conform to specified standards for 'weight, figure, straight teeth, complexion, facial regularity'.

I have discussed in a previous article (Purcell 1989) how gender is both an attribute which employees bring to the workplace and a process which they experience as part of employment. Interactive service jobs in hospitality, tourism and leisure exemplify occupations where gender (and indeed, sexuality) are explicit aspects of the job. Kinnaird and Hall (1994: 210) have discussed how tourism is gendered in four distinct ways: gendered tourists, gendered hosts, gendered tourism marketing and gendered tourism products. Sexuality comes most forcefully into the last of these two categories, where women are used to promote and to be part of the tourism product as, for example, in airline advertising.

Gender relations in tourism and hospitality reflect wider social gender relations. For example, it is no accident that sex tourism has been particularly successful *in* (and appeals particularly to men *from*) socially gender-segregated cultures where the sexes lead very different lives, in terms of social roles and access to the public sphere, where women have traditionally been required to be subservient to men (Hall 1994). As Badger (1993: 4) has pointed out in relation to tourism marketing in general, both client and host countries have allowed women to be treated as a commodity. Air stewardesses dressed in slinky, low-cut dresses to serve champagne to Australian business-class travellers as part of the internal flight 'Gold lamé service' (Williams 1988), or 'bunny girls', working for

Playboy International, are particularly blatant examples on this continuum which ranges from the 'attractive' theme park canteen assistants and chambermaids sought by the organizations researched by Adkins to sex-workers in clubs and on the streets.

Adkins' and Filby's research reveals that women employed in most interactive service jobs are expected to package and present themselves in 'gender-appropriate' ways, where their sexuality is an implicit – sometimes explicit – aspect of their work role. Both refer to the requirement to 'take' sexually explicit teasing and flirtation from male customers (and sometimes colleagues) as 'part of the job' (cf. Adkins 1995: 130). Filby (1992: 29) discusses how:

> talk is the main way in which 'sex' and 'sexuality' are constituted in the workplace [but] sexuality is also embodied in gaze, deportment and clothing, and sometimes in more obviously expressive encounters. Of interest in the present context, however, is the extent to which these moments are related to the milieu of service delivery as implicitly constructed by management, a milieu which is envisaged as an aid to business.

Pringle (1989) has observed that sexualized interaction between men and women at work (where men tend to be in higher status occupations) tends explicitly to draw attention to female sexuality and implicitly enhance male confidence and sexual identity. This is clearly the effect on (male) customers and clients that employers are looking for when they specify that women service workers should conform to 'height for weight' and 'attractiveness' criteria.

In one sense, this illustrates Urry's (1990) observation that such commercial services involve the sale of an experience, where the quality of the social interaction, including the visual presentation of interactive service workers, is an intrinsic part of the service itself. In another, stronger, sense, as argued by Adkins (1995: 146–7),

> women are thus not only expected to be 'economically productive' but also 'sexually productive' workers. The fact that it was only women who were required to carry out sexual servicing as a condition of their employment shows that men and women participated in the two workplaces within substantially different relations of production.

In many workplaces and resorts, the sexualized and leisure-focused ambience can lead to volatility. The line between sexual banter and sexual harassment is drawn differently by different people and the industry has been alleged to be prone to sexual harassment (Beck 1986; Eller 1990; Woods and Kavanaugh 1994). The structure of the industry and the combination of sociability and long hours of work has been found to put an enormous strain on marriages and be conducive to extra-marital affairs (*Caterer and Hotelkeeper* 1994: 79). On the other hand, this negative tendency also highlights the positive attractions of even low-paid hospitality and tourism employment; the fact that it provides scope for *fun*. Adkins concedes (1995: 154) that the women she observed, while on balance constrained by sexualized interaction, did in fact enjoy some of it. Sexual harassment and much 'sexualized' banter in the workplace, however, has been observed to be more about controlling women than about celebrating their sexuality (see Thomas and Kitzinger 1994, for a recent summary of the debate).

Sex-typed jobs, in this narrower sense, distort the operation of the labour market, in that they not only preclude the appointment of males, but also most potential female applicants, because they are actually 'sexuality-typed', not simply sex-typed: they 'require' only certain kinds – shapes, sizes and ages – of women. In one sense, this is Rousseau's 'natural inequalities' (Dahrendorf 1968: 154) being used to structure 'social inequalities', but it is not entirely clear in which direction the advantage operates. Such job recruitment reinforces the tyranny of gender stereotypes, which constrain both male and female behaviour and opportunities. Research on the relationship between researcher and employer-rated attractiveness and earnings suggests that there is evidence of a tendency on the part of employers to discriminate in favour of 'attractive' and against 'less attractive' candidates for jobs and promotions (Hamermesh and Biddle 1994). Although evaluations of beauty and attractiveness are, of course, subjective and vary among different cultures and within cultures over time, research findings indicate a remarkable degree of consistency and stability within given cultures, with stronger reactions (both positive and negative) to women's appearance than to men's (Hatfield and Sprecher 1986).

PATRIARCHALLY PRESCRIBED OCCUPATIONS

The final gendered category of occupations is those which are prescribed by patriarchal precepts. The social dynamics which reinforce recruitment to and exclusion from these occupations encourage women to be nurturers and men to be patriarchs. They encourage women to 'be mum' socially, in taking responsibility for housekeeping in hotels or guest houses; they encourage women to be dependent on men by providing opportunities for 'component waged' jobs (Siltanen 1994) which the HCTC (1994: 37) note, without irony, 'appeal to women who wish to combine the opportunity to earn an income with their domestic responsibilities'. At the extreme, they provide feudal opportunities for women to work as 'unpaid family workers' (Sly 1994: 413) – sometimes for multinational organizations: a strange anachronism in post-industrial societies.

Such 'family production' is taken to its apotheosis in small businesses – small hotels, guesthouses, pubs, clubs, cafés – where husband and wife teams work together, with the woman frequently employed as 'unpaid family worker' (Goffee and Scase; 1983; Urry 1990). It has long been established that women's unpaid labour in such enterprises has been crucial to their survival and success, but Adkins' (1995: 72 ff.) research revealed that such practices are not confined to small, autonomous operations but are also characteristic of large multidivisional (sometimes multinational) organizations in the hotel, restaurant and licensed trade industries. Companies were found to advertise for 'couples' and 'manager with spouse to assist' but further investigation revealed that in such cases, although work was explicitly required of both partners, the employment contracts operated between the husbands and the companies. The wives' labour was thus subsumed within their husbands', rendering them dependants whose maintenance and subsistence, no less than non-employed wives, was contingent upon the goodwill of their partners, who controlled their labour.

Company representatives interviewed by Adkins extolled the virtues of such arrangements: reduced labour costs (normally two for the price of one-and-a-quarter times a single manager's wage), reliability, stability, good coverage of the range of administrative, domestic and affective aspects of the job plus, as one respondent put it, '[Men] like to be served by women. . . . We like to employ couples because of the custom that wives generate' (ibid.: 90); an example, in Adkins' terms, of 'sexual exchange value' and/or sex-typed expectations of nurturing inherent in much 'women's' work. One company which had attempted to restructure by phasing out such contracts had encountered opposition from managers and increased costs and operational difficulties which had persuaded them to return to recruiting married couples. Adkins' interviews with managers and wives in such partnerships suggested that the normal division of labour was for men to 'front' the operation and women to provide the domestic servicing, housekeeping and support stereotypically reminiscent of 'traditional' breadwinner/homemaker conjugal divisions of labour. Her underlying analysis draws attention to the fact that such employment arrangements are particularly transparent examples of how male labour power is often not only underpinned, to a greater or lesser extent, by the unpaid labour of wives, but of how such unpaid labour is assumed, by employers, as an inherent part of the male contribution.

Hospitality industry employment, and tourism-related activity in particular, especially in relatively remote peripheral tourism locations, is also characterized by a high proportion of self-employment, family-owned businesses, the employment of women, part-time employment and small-scale, seasonal operations employing few people (Medlik 1989). In 1992, over 12 per cent of employees in the commercial sector of the industry were estimated to be self-employed (HCTC 1994) and 60 per cent of establishments were owned or operated by self-employed people. Census of Employment figures indicate that 87 per cent of hotels and 92 per cent of restaurants employed between one and ten employees in 1991 (HCTC 1994: 24). Some types of family businesses fall within the category of 'patriarchally prescribed' employment, in that the women's male partners maintain control over both the type and extent of the work which women undertake within the enterprise and the income which is obtained from it.

Breathnach et al.'s (1994) study of tourism in Ireland illustrates an alternative form of control over women's access to work. They estimated (ibid.: 96) that for each approved bed-and-breakfast enterprise in the locality they researched, there were three unapproved. They identified the impact of ecclesiastical patriarchy in discouraging women's employment and, paradoxically, underpinning such informal economic activity, commenting that: 'It is clear that many women remain outside the paid workforce due to the traditional social and cultural value systems of the Roman Catholic Church'(ibid.: 58). As well as being more compatible with domestic responsibilities, it is more socially acceptable for women in such subcultures to earn money by work carried on within the household than to take a job in the public domain.

However, other types of self-employment challenge patriarchal control by providing women with control over the types and extent of the work which they undertake and the earnings which they gain from it. Ireland (1993) carried out a fascinating analysis of inter-generational gender and class relations in relation to tourism, in Sennen, a Cornish seaside resort. He traces women's involvement as 'markers of the boundaries between locals and visitors' (ibid.: 673) as bed-and-breakfast and guesthouse landladies, from the late nine-teenth century onwards – providing an economic contribution to an otherwise declining economy where the traditional mainstay had been the fishing industry. He provides a vivid picture of male resentment on the part of host husbands whose lives were dis-rupted, though their households may have been kept solvent by the tourists, and of an industry run by women who, although they tended to maintain a public image of gender subordination, were nevertheless empowered by their capacity to earn, which endowed them with private control within the household (ibid.: 670). It is clear from this study that, despite a perception that men participated more than their fathers had done in the work generated by bed-and-breakfast activities, in fact the reality of men's contribution has been exaggerated; a not infrequent finding in studies of household divi-sions of labour. All of these women were in effect self-employed, as individuals or in household partnerships, with many ambiguously situated at the edge of the 'informal economy'.

ACCESS TO CAREERS IN THE SECTOR

The construction of well-paid breadwinner jobs in hospitality and tourism as 'men's jobs' and the consequent virtual exclusion of women from such jobs and their concentration in low-paid and part-time jobs, reinforces women's subordination and economic dependency. But is there any evidence that, in this industry which is numerically dominated by women, equal opportunities legislation has made any impact in recent years? Crompton and Sanderson (1989) commented on the increasing importance of professional credentials in the hospitality industry and hypothesized that, although women have historically been largely excluded from senior management in the industry, their considerably greater numbers on relevant vocational higher education courses might lead to increasing female penetration of career occupations. Pre-vious research (HCITB 1987) indicated that female degree and diploma-holding entrants to the industry are considerably less likely than their male counterparts to embark on a career trajectory designed to lead them into mainstream management, and that initial inequalities of access are reinforced by subsequent early career moves.

Research carried out in 1993 (Purcell 1994; Purcell and Quinn 1995) reinforces the earlier findings. An alumni study of 712 degree and HND students who completed hotel and catering management courses at 30 UK educational institutions in 1989 revealed that women were:

- less likely than men to have been given the opportunity to develop supervisory or management skills as part of their under-graduate industrial placements;
- more likely than men to have had difficulty in obtaining suitable employment;
- less likely than men to have developed careers in the industry;
- less likely than men to have been given the opportunity to acquire recognized post-experience qualifications;
- more likely than men to be underachieving professionally;
- less likely than men to perceive that they had 'a great deal of autonomy' in their current employment;
- less likely than men to have a strong possibility of promotion in their current employment;
- more likely than men to express dissatisfaction with their career to date.

The most unambiguous indications of persistent obstacles to equal opportunities were the differentials in rewards. The average salary of the highly qualified women in this cohort who were employed in the hospitality industry at the time of the survey in 1993, more than three years after graduation, was £11,562, whereas the average salary for their male peers was £14,816. These differentials were reinforced by differences in fringe benefits, with men in the com-mercial hospitality sector significantly more likely than women to be entitled to valuable 'perks' such as company cars, free or subsidized meals, low cost housing, private health insurance, com-pany share ownership schemes and product discounts. Rubery and Fagan (1993: 102) have pointed out that women managers in hotels and catering earn below average wages for *women* as a whole, quite apart from being well below average in relation to *managers'* wages.

These findings suggest that highly qualified women in Hotel and Catering Management have different experiences of early career development than their male counterparts. They are more likely to have had negative experience in their supervised work experience year, more likely to have difficulty in obtaining the kind of job they want, less likely to have jobs which offer them intrinsic satisfaction and good career prospects and finally, less likely to have 'professional' salaries with accompanying fringe benefits. The 'qualification lever' seems to have been somewhat less effective then Crompton and Sanderson predicted.

The fact that hotel management is a notoriously 'greedy occupation' which requires long working hours, willingness to be geographically mobile and where the boundaries between work and non-work are difficult to draw is often referred to by managers, including women themselves, as a disincentive to women (Hicks 1990, *Caterer and Hotelkeeper* 1994: 79–80). What Guerrier (1986) has called these *formal* aspects of male exclusionary practice, the way that jobs and working hours are constructed, are reinforced by the *informal* aspects – the 'old boy' network of informal recruitment practices circumscribed by prejudice and stereotyped thinking, which discourages women and encourages men to apply for career advancement. Recent research among managers (Hicks 1990, Walsh and McKenna 1991, Berkeley-Scott 1991) has unearthed profoundly sexist attitudes among senior managers, most of whom appear to exhibit all the characteristics of a strong and self-perpetuating occupational community. There was much evidence of an unshakeable belief in the particular ('male') characteristics required to be a successful operational manager in the hospitality industry, alongside stereotypical beliefs about women's attributes and orientations to work (Hicks 1990: 353–8), particularly their supposed weaknesses as managers. Women were believed to be insufficiently tough and lacking in leadership qualities (especially the ability to take responsibility and to manage men). In addition, they were believed to have an (unsubstantiated) propensity to have higher turnover rates; and customers were alleged to expect (and by implication prefer) that a man should be in charge (Walsh and McKenna 1991: 5). Hicks' detailed analysis of the non-verbal responses and the language which managers used to talk about their work and their understandings about why there are so few women managers in the industry is particularly revealing of the informal barriers to equality of opportunity and the different expectations held of highly qualified male and female recruits to the industry. These beliefs derive from a gendered ideology and they inform and reinforce recruitment to and exclusion from what I have labelled 'patriarchally prescribed' occupations in the industry, with the effect of excluding most women.

CONCLUSION

There are thus three conceptually distinct determinants of gendered recruitment, work and employment within tourism-related accommodation and catering services: employers' economic rationality, the significance of sexuality in gendered demand for labour and the persistence of patriarchal relations and ideology. Their distribution as explanatory variables varies among occupations, and while it makes sense to talk about mutually reinforcing pressures exerted by capitalism and gender relations, the relationships between capitalism and sexuality and between patriarchy and sexuality are complex, in that pleasure and exploitation may be two sides of the same coin. To recognize that women for whom there is a sex-typed element to their work are vulnerable to exploitation is not to deny that such work may be considerably more attractive to them (and enjoyable) than some of the alternative gender-contingent (or indeed, gender-neutral) jobs that may be available to them. Pringle's (1988) analysis of secretaries draws attention to this paradox of undervalued women (in economic terms) deriving value and pleasure from the sex-typed appreciation of bosses and clients to a degree that made it difficult to define them as exploited victims.

In many tourism-related jobs, the boundaries between work, leisure and social relationships which give meaning to the human condition are obscured by the industry's focus on pleasure: giving pleasure and facilitating enjoyment. The Project on Disney (1995: 141), while reporting restricted, highly prescribed and often humiliating working conditions, invariably reported employees liking the work itself: the people and 'being part of the Disney magic'. Marshall (1986) similarly described the positive orientations to work of low-paid catering workers in Scotland who experienced their work as socially fulfilling. Good working relationships, the *frisson* of flirtations in largely safe public arenas and the carnival atmosphere of the leisure industry, geared to facilitating 'good times' for its clients, may not be adequate substitutes for good pay and contractual employment rights and, on analysis, may not counterbalance the negative effects of stereotyping on restricting opportunities, but they may go some way to explaining why sex-typed occupations survive and continue to attract job applicants as well as customers.

BIBLIOGRAPHY

Adkins, L. (1995) *Gendered work: sexuality, family and the labour market*, Milton Keynes: Open University Press.

Bacon, W. and K. Lewis (1990) 'Sex Changes', *Leisure Management*, vol. 10, no. 10: 31–2.

Badger, A. (1993) 'Why not acknowledge women?', *In Focus*, no. 10, Winter: 2–5.

Bagguley, P. (1991) 'The Patriarchal Restructuring of Gender Segregation: A Case Study of the Hotel and Catering Industry', *Sociology*, vol. 25, no. 4: 607–25.

Bagguley, P. (1990) 'Gender and Labour Flexibility in Hotel and Catering, *Service Industry Journal*, vol. 10, no. 4: 737–47.

Baum, T. (1993) *Human Resource Issues in International Tourism*, Oxford: Butterworth Heinemann.

Beck, J. (1986), 'Developing Women Managers in the Hotel and Catering Industry', *Women in Management Review*, Spring: 31–7.

Beechey, V. (1987), *Unequal Work*, London: Verso.

Berkeley Scott (1991) *The Hotel, Catering and Leisure Business Review*, London: Berkeley Scott and Marketpower.

Breathnach, P. Henry, M. Drea, S. and M. O'Flaherty (1994) 'Gender in Irish Tourism Employment', in V. Kinnaird and D. Hall (eds) *Tourism: A Gender Analysis*, Chichester: John Wiley.

Bruegel, I. (1982) 'Women as a reserve army of labour: a note on the recent British experience' in E. Whitelegg (ed.) *The Changing Experience of Women*, Oxford: Martin Robertson.

Butler, R.W. (1994) 'Seasonality in tourism: issues and problems' in A.V. Seaton (ed.) *Tourism: the State of the Art*, Chichester: John Wiley.

Caterer and Hotelkeeper (1992) 'Women must fight men for top jobs', 21 May: 14.

Caterer and Hotelkeeper (1994) 'Married to the Job?', 10 February: 79–80.

Chivers, T.S. (1973) 'The Proletarianisation of a service worker ' *Sociological Review*, 21: 633–56.

CIR (Commission on Industrial Relations) (1971) *The Hotel and Catering Industry*, London: HMSO.

Crompton, R. and Sanderson K. (1990) *Gendered Jobs and Social Change*, London: Unwin Hyman.

Department of Employment (1971) *Manpower Studies no. 10: Hotels*, London: HMSO.

Dahrendorf, R. (1968) 'The origin of inequality' in *Essays in the Theory of Society*, London: Routledge and Kegan Paul.

Davidson, M. and Cooper, C. (1992) *Shattering the Glass Ceiling: The Woman Manager*, London: Paul Chapman Publishing.

DE (Department of Employment) (1987) 'Jobs in tourism: note by the Department of Employment', *Employment Gazette*, July: 336.

Davidson, M. and Cooper, C. (1983) *Stress and the Woman Manager*, London: Martin Robertson.

Eller, M.E. (1990) 'Sexual harassment in the hotel industry: the need to focus on prevention', *Hospitality Research Journal*, vol. 14, no. 2: 431–40.

ETB/IMS (English Tourist Board/Institute of Manpower Studies) (1986) *Jobs in Tourism and Leisure: A Labour Market Review*, London and Falmer: ETB/IMS.

European Commission (1994) *Employment in Europe*, COM (94)381, Brussels: CEC: Directorate General for Employment, Industrial Relations and Social Affairs.

Filby, M. (1992) ''The figures, the personality and the bums': service work and sexuality', *Work, Employment and Society*, vol. 6, no. 2: 23–42.

Flogenfeldt, T. (1988) 'The employment paradox in seasonal tourism', paper presented at Pre-Congress Meeting of International Geographical Union, Christchurch, New Zealand.

Gabriel, Y. (1988) *Working Lives in Catering*, London: Routledge and Kegan Paul.

Gershuny, J., Godwin, M., and Jones, S. (1994) 'The Domestic Labour Revolution: a Process of Lagged Adaptation' in M. Anderson, F. Bechhofer and J. Gershuny (eds) *The Social and Political Economy of the Household*, Oxford: Oxford University Press.

Guerrier, Y. (1986) 'Hotel management: an unsuitable job for a woman?', *Service Industries Journal*, vol. 6, no. 2: 227–40.

Goffee, R. and R. Scase (1983) 'Class, entrepreneurship and the service sector: towards a conceptual clarification', *Service Industries Journal*, vol. 3, no. 2: 146–60.

Hall, C.M. (1994) 'Gender and economic interests in tourism prostitution: the nature, development and complications of sex tourism in South-East Asia' in V. Kinnaird and D. Hall (eds) *Tourism: a Gender Analysis*, Chichester: John Wiley.

Hamermesh, D.S., and Biddle, J.E., (1994) 'Beauty and the labour market', *The American Economic Review*, vol. 84, no. 5: 1174–94.

Hatfield, E., and Sprecher, S. (1986), '*Mirror, mirror . . . the importance of looks in every day life*', Albany, NY: State University of New York Press.

Hennessey, S. (1994) 'Female employment in tourism development in South-West England', in V. Kinnaird and D. Hall, *Tourism and Gender Analysis*, Chichester: John Wiley.

Hennessey, S. Shaw, G. and A. Williams (1986) *The role of tourism in local economies: a pilot study of Looe, Cornwall*, Exeter: University of Exeter.

Hey, V. (1986) *Patriarchy and Pub Culture*, London: Tavistock.

Hicks, L. (1990) 'Excluded Women: How can this Happen in the Hotel World?', *The Service Industries Journal*, vol. 10, no. 2: 348–63.

Hochschild, A. (1983) *The Managed Heart*, Berkeley and Los Angeles: University of California Press.

Horwath and Horwath (1988) 'Human resources – the most important issue facing hoteliers', *Hospitality*, November, no. 94: 7.

HOST Consultancy (1991) *Jobs in Tourism and Leisure: A Labour Market Review*, London: English Tourist Board.

HCITB (Hotel and Catering Industry Training Board) (1984) *Women's Path to Management in the Hotel and Catering Industry*, London: HCITB.

HCITB (1987) *Women in the Hotel and Catering Industry*, London: HCTB.

HCTC (Hotel and Catering Industry Training Company) (1994) *Catering and Hospitality Industry – Key: Facts and Figures Research Report 1994*, London: HCTC.

IER (1994) *Review of Economy and Employment, Occupational Assessment*, University of Warwick: Institute for Employment Research.

Ireland, M. (1993) 'Gender and Class Relations in Tourism Employment', *Annals of Tourism Research*, vol., 20 no. 4: 666–84.

Johnston, K. (1985) 'Labour Turnover in Hotels Revisited', *The Service Industries Journal*, vol. 5, no. 2: 135–52.

Jones, M. (1992) 'Failure to promote women "a serious loss"', *Caterer and Hotelkeeper*, 9 January: 12.

Kinnaird, K. and D. Hall (1994) *Tourism: a Gender Analysis*, Chichester: John Wiley.

Leidner, R. (1993) *Fast Food, Fast Talk*, Berkeley and Los Angeles: University of California Press.

Lovering, J. (1994) 'Employers, the sex-typing of jobs, and economic restructuring', in A. Scott (ed.) *Gender Segregation and Social Change*, Oxford: Oxford University Press.

Lucas, R. (1993) 'Hospitality industry employment: emerging trends', *International Journal of Contemporary Hospitality*, vol. 5, no. 5: 23–6.

Marshall, G. (1986) 'the workplace culture of a licensed restaurant', *Theory, Culture and Society*, vol. 3, no. 1: 33–47.

Medlik, S. (1989) *Tourism Employment in Wales*, Cardiff: Wales Tourist Board.

Metcalf, H. (1987) *Employment Structures in Tourism and Leisure*, IMS Report no. 143, Brighton: Institute for Manpower Studies, University of Sussex.

NEDO (National Economic Development Council) (1992) *UK Tourism: Competing for Growth, Report by the National Development Council's Working Party on Competitiveness in Tourism and Hospitality*, London: NEDO.

Novarra, V. (1980) *Men's Work, Women's Work*, London: Marion Boyars.

Parsons, D. (1992) 'Developments in the UK tourism and leisure labour market', in R. Lindley (ed.) *Women's Employment: Britain in the Single European Market*, London: Equal Opportunities Commission, HMSO.

Parsons, D. and Cave, P. (1991) *Developing Managers for Tourism*, London: NEDO.

Phillips, A. and Taylor, B. (1980) 'Sex and skill: notes towards a feminist economics', *Feminist Review*, no. 6: 79–88.

Price, L. (1994) 'Poor personnel practice in the hotel and catering industry: does it matter?', *Human Resource Management Journal*, vol. 4, no. 4: 44–62.

Pringle, R. (1988) *Secretaries Talk: Sexuality, Power and Work*, London: Verso.

Project on Disney (1995) *Inside the Mouse: Work and Play at Disney World*, Durham and London: Duke University Press.

Purcell, K. (1989) 'Gender at Work' in D. Gallie (ed.) *Employment in Britain*, Oxford: Blackwell.

Purcell, K. (1994) 'Equal opportunity in the hospitality industry: custom and credentials', *International Journal of Hospitality Management*, vol. 2: 2: 127–40.

Purcell, K. and J. Quinn (1995) *Hospitality Management Education and Employment Trajectories*, Oxford: Oxford Brookes University.

Rees, G. and S. Fielder (1992) 'The services economy, subcontracting and the new employment relations: contract catering and cleaning' *Employment and Society*, vol. 6, no. 3: 347–68.

Riley, M. (1991) 'An analysis of hotel labour markets' in C.P. Cooper (ed.) *Progress in Tourism, Recreation and Hospitality Management*, London: Belhaven Press.

Rubery, J. and C. Fagan (1993) *Occupational Segregation of Women and Men in the European Community*, Social Europe Supplement 3/93, Brussels: CEC, Directorate General for Employment, Industrial and Social Affairs.

Scott, A. (1995) *Gender Segregation and Social Change*, Oxford: Oxford University Press.

Sharpe, S., (1976) *'Just Like a Girl': How Girls Learn to be Women*, Harmondsworth: Penguin.

Siltanen, J. (1994), *Locating Gender*, London: UCL Press.

Smith, A.D. (1986) 'Miscellaneous services' in A.D. Smith (ed.) *Commercial Service Industries*, Aldershot: Gower Press.

Spradley, J. and B. Mann (1975) *The Cocktail Waitress: Women's Work in a Man's World*, New York: John Wiley.

Sly, F. (1994) 'Mothers in the labour market', *Employment Gazette*, November: 403–13.

Thomas, A. and C. Kitzinger (1994) ' "It's just something that happens": the invisibility of sexual harassment in the workplace', *Gender, Work and Organisation*, vol. 1, no. 3: 151–61.

Urry, J. (1990) *The Tourist Gaze: Leisure and Travel in Contemporary Societies*, London: Sage.

Walsh, M.E. and McKenna, M. (1991) 'Women – the under-utilised resource in tourism employment', *Tourism*, September: 5.

Walsh T.J. (1991) 'Flexible employment in the Retail and Hotel Trades', in A. Pollert (ed.) *Farewell to Flexibility?*, Oxford: Basil Blackwell.

Walsh, T. J. (1989) 'Part-time employment and labour market policies', *National Westminster Bank Quarterly Review*, May: 43–55 .

Watson, G. (1992) 'Hours of work in Great Britain and Europe: endemic from the UK and European labour force surveys' *Employment Gazette*, November: 539–57.

White (1988) 'Women in leisure service management' in E. Wimbush and M. Talbot (eds) *Relative Freedoms*, Milton Keynes: Open University Press.

Whyte, W. F. (1949) 'The social structure of the restaurant', *American Journal of Sociology*, vol. 54: 302–10.

Williams, C. (1988) *Blue, White and Pink Collar Workers: Technicians, Bank Employees and Flight Attendants*, London: Allen and Unwin.

Wood, R. (1992) *Working in Hotels and Catering*, London: Routledge.

Wood, R. (1989) 'Hospitality industry labour trends: British and international experiences', *Tourism Management*, September: 297–306.

Woods and Kavanaugh (1994) 'Gender discrimination and sexual harassment as experienced by hospitality industry managers', *The Cornell Hotel and Restaurant Administration Quarterly*, February: 16–21.

Chapter 4

Chances and choices
Women and tourism in Northern Cyprus

Julie Scott

INTRODUCTION

Numerous studies on tourism have concluded that men and women do not benefit equally from tourism development in their communities (Harvey *et al.* 1995). In the countries of Western Europe and northern America, tourism, and in particular the hotel sector, is usually regarded as a 'feminized' industry (OECD 1988: 21). In many developing countries, in contrast, men tend to predominate in large-scale, 'capitalist' hotels, especially when tourism is the main economic activity of the area (Bryden 1973; Boissevain and Inglott 1979; Smaoui 1979). Women's access to tourism jobs often depends on there being other, more remunerative, sources of employment available to men; frequently excluded from all but the most menial work (Reynoso y Valle and de Regt 1979; Samarasuriya 1982), women also suffer from a continuing 'gender-based salary gap' (Harvey *et al.* 1995: 363). The relative benefits of tourism development to women and men reflect local norms concerning the sexual division of labour. At the same time, it has been argued, women's subordinate position in the tourism employment hierarchy both reflects and reinforces the gendered imagery and stereotyping which is associated with, in particular, sun, sea and sand tourism (as shown by Margaret Marshment's chapter in this book; see also Castelberg-Koulma 1991; Swain 1995).

Small-scale and family-run businesses have been found to offer greater and more varied employment to women than large, luxury hotels and restaurants (Reynoso y Valle and de Regt 1979); and involvement in the small business sector, in contrast to conventional large-scale tourism development, is often regarded as having the potential to empower women. Taking paying guests into the home frequently fits into a pre-existing gender division of household labour and responsibilities which enables women to retain control of a business seen as an extension of their domestic duties (Bouquet 1982; Hermans 1983; Kousis 1989; Garcia-Ramon et al. 1995). Women can also gain confidence and prestige from their ability to make a financial contribution to household resources, as well as from their contact with visitors and organizations from 'outside' (Bouquet 1984; Ireland 1993; Castelberg-Koulma 1991; Garcia-Ramon et al. 1995). A strong role for women in small-scale local tourism development can provide the basis for collective action by women in pursuit of common interests (Armstrong 1977) and can promote alternatives to the stereotypical images of women as holi-day sexual fantasy (Castelberg-Koulma 1991). Women's role in the small-scale tourism sector is associated with tourism alternatives in other ways too, as a result both of the generally low capital-intensity of women's businesses (Hermans 1983) and their involvement with rural and farm tourism as sustainable alternatives to sun, sea and sand tourism (Repena-Osolnik 1983; Bouquet 1982; Castelberg-Koulma 1991; Garcia-Ramon et al. 1995).

In this chapter I examine the case of a developing tourism industry in which, contrary to what might be expected, women play a marginal role in small-scale family-run hotel businesses, and on the whole fare better in larger establishments with a more formal and bureaucratic employment structure; and I consider the implications of this case for understanding gendered perspectives on and experiences of tourism. I argue that whilst tourism employment is 'overtly gender biased, reflecting local and trans-national norms of "women's work"' (Swain 1995: 250), the female labour force, which is often implicitly treated as an undifferentiated input, is in fact highly diverse, as is the range of tourism employment available; and that this diversity has to be part of explanations which attempt to account for tourism development's impacts on locally constructed gender roles and relationships.

The cases are taken from research carried out over eighteen months in a sea-side town on the northern coast of Cyprus.[1] The main methods were participant observation; semi-structured and open-ended interviews with both men and women (about 100 individuals in total) working in a wide range of tourism activities; and a systematic survey of three local newspapers. The more formal interviews were carried out by prior arrangement, sometimes in the place of work and sometimes outside working hours in the interviewee's home. In some cases the interviewees were part of a family or neighbourhood network with whom I had social contact; in other cases, managers selected individuals from a variety of departments on the basis of who was free at any given time, and made space available in which the interviews could take place. The initial contact with owners and managers of tourism businesses was usually made 'cold' – i.e. I walked in off the street and asked for cooperation with my research – or with the help of an intermediary. The social context in which these interviews took place often meant that they turned into group discussions, with colleagues, customers, neighbours or other family members of both sexes joining in, and interviews commonly lasted anything from 20 minutes to one or two hours or more. In addition, some of the themes presented here emerged and were pursued in the course of everyday interaction and conversation in a variety of social settings. A weakness of the data is that I was not able to interview women who did not actively participate in the family business and who were not present in the premises where the business was carried out. Whilst the incidence of non-participation by women in the family tourism business is in itself an important indicator of the trends which I examine below, I have no qualitative data concerning these individual women's decisions not to work in the business other than the explanations offered by husbands and the comments and suggestions made by other female informants.

In this chapter I start by examining Northern Cyprus's tourism development against the background of Turkish Cypriots' condi- tions before 1974 and the political and economic consequences of the division of the island. I then discuss women's position in Turkish Cypriot society and the characteristics of the female work- force, before going on to look at the market, resources and employ- ment in a range of accommodation businesses in the town of Girne (Kyrenia).[2]

TOURISM IN NORTHERN CYPRUS

Cyprus was partitioned in 1974 following a *coup d'état* engineered by the military government of Greece and subsequent military intervention by Turkey. With the exchange of populations which took place during the following year, the north of the island became a Turkish Cypriot area and the south Greek Cypriot. The division of the island was a painful and traumatic experience for both Greek and Turkish Cypriots (Loizos 1981); but whereas partition has never been accepted as permanent or legitimate by Greek Cypriots, Turkish Cypriot policy has been to consolidate their position and establish a viable state in the north. Tourism presented itself as a natural development strategy. Cyprus had 'taken off' as a tourist destination in the late 1960s (Ioannides 1992). Most of the pre-1974 tourism development had occurred in the north of the island, and approximately 65 per cent of total bed capacity, mostly concentrated in the resorts of Girne (Kyrenia) and Mağusa (Famagusta), was left in the area under Turkish and Turkish Cypriot control. Of the total 10,200 licensed beds in these two resorts, 6,000 were in the Mağusa suburb of Maraş (Varosha) which, up to the time of writing, has remained a closed area under military control (Lockhart and Ashton 1990). With only a few exceptions, the touristic establishments in the north were Greek Cypriot or foreign owned. Before 1974, Turkish Cypriot participation in tourism development had been minimal, a result of the geographical confinement and economic immiseration of the majority of Turkish Cypriots during the inter-communal conflicts of the 1960s and early 1970s (Purcell 1969; Ladbury and King 1982; Berner 1992), and of formal and informal discrimination against would-be Turkish Cypriot investors (Çağın 1990; Martin 1993).

Despite its losses, Greek Cypriot tourism has made a rapid recovery since 1974, developing new resorts in the south and attracting more than a million visitors in 1988 (Lockhart and Ashton 1990). In the north, too, tourism development has been prioritized as the 'locomotive sector of the economy', but with markedly less success. The major obstacle to its tourism is the 'illegal' status of the north. The 'Turkish Republic of Northern Cyprus' was unilaterally declared in 1983, but is currently recognized only by Turkey. The air and seaports of Northern Cyprus are deemed illegal points of entry to the island, and a civil aviation boycott on flights to Northern Cyprus means that aeroplanes must touch down in Turkey before continuing to the Turkish Cypriot airport at Ercan. A similar boycott exists on foreign investment in Northern Cyprus and, until recently, it was virtually impossible to publicize Northern Cyprus as a tourist destination in European countries. As a result, Turkish Cypriot tourism is heavily dependent on Turkey, both for financial support and as a tourist market and gateway to the rest of the world. Although the number of licensed beds in the north has slowly crept up to a total of about 7,000 (in

1992), bed occupancy rates have never exceeded 50 per cent, and seldom more than 35 per cent; for seven of the last seventeen years up to 1992 they have been below 25 per cent (SPO 1981–1992).

Roughly 80 per cent of all tourists are Turkish, many of these 'luggage tourists' who are commissioned by Turkish retailers to make bulk purchases of those items which are available more cheaply in Northern Cyprus for resale in Turkey: such tourists tend to stay only two or three nights, in cheap and often unlicensed *pansiyon* (boarding house) accommodation. Tourists from countries other than Turkey constituted only 17–25 per cent of total arrivals throughout the 1980s; in contrast, most visitors to the south of the island come from Western Europe, with about 30 per cent coming from the UK. In 1987, tourist arrivals to the north totalled 185,000, compared with 1,000,000 to the south.

Turkish Cypriot tourism began to experience something of a boom in the late 1980s, largely as a result of the more proactive tourism policy adopted by the government, and investment by the London-based Polly Peck conglomerate owned by the Turkish Cypriot businessman Asil Nadir. His introduction of charter flights from the UK raised the numbers of European tourists to Northern Cyprus and stimulated further hotel construction. The planned target of 250,600 tourists by 1992 was exceeded in 1989; 24 per cent of these tourists were non-Turkish. However, the Gulf War of 1990, and the collapse of Polly Peck later that year, brought an abrupt end to this upward trend. Businesses which had borrowed heavily at high interest rates to take advantage of the short-lived boom found themselves on the verge of bankruptcy. Only in 1993, when Kurdish bombing campaigns in Turkish resorts made some operators transfer their bookings to Northern Cyprus, did tourism again begin to pick up.

The pattern of tourism development in Northern Cyprus has, therefore, been perilous and unsteady. Whilst it provides a considerable share of invisible earnings, as a proportion of GDP it has remained static at around 2 per cent, and agriculture, in particular citrus production, remains the backbone of the economy. However, the agricultural sector, too, is beset with problems, resulting largely from marketing bottlenecks and high inflation (Morvaridi 1993). With the lion's share of resources earmarked for tourism development, agricultural activity has been increasingly marginalized.[3]

The tourist market is fragmented, each segment having substantially different expectations of Northern Cyprus as a tourist destination, as well as requiring different channels of communication and types of business relationship for marketing and sales purposes. Turkish tourists (including luggage tourists) predominate, accompanied by a small but growing number of European tourists. Many of these are higher income older couples and families, travelling with small and special interest tour operators who market Northern Cyprus as 'the last unspoilt corner of the Mediterranean', and it is from this group that a demand for 'authentic' village tourism has begun to make itself felt. So far, however, there has been little in the way of organized response, and it is largely the foreign (mostly British and German) leaseholders of restored village properties in the picturesque mountain villages around Girne who have capitalized on this demand by letting out their holiday homes during those times of the year when they are not themselves in residence.[4] For the majority of Turkish Cypriots, the image of the *köy* (village), with its associations of the backward and parochial, does not accord with the island's tourism image, and tourism development policy continues to prioritize the construction of purpose-built hotels and holiday villages more suitable to the mainstream mass tourism market.

WOMEN AND WORK IN NORTHERN CYPRUS

Twenty years ago, very few Turkish Cypriot women worked outside the home. Those who did were generally the educated daughters of affluent families working in urban professional occupations (Ladbury 1979). Not only were there few educational and economic opportunities to enable the majority of women to take up paid employment: they were also constrained by notions of 'respectability', embodied in the concept of *namus* (reputation or sexual honour/shame). Both a woman's marriage prospects and the reputation of her menfolk depended on avoiding situations which might give rise to gossip, and this entailed restrictions on women's business activities, employment and social contacts outside the home (ibid.).

Women's employment has increased dramatically in the intervening twenty years, as a result of the expansion in their educational and employment opportunities, and a relaxation in the code of reputation, permitting greater freedom to women outside the home. Young women generally expect to go out to work, even after having children; and working outside the home has also become an option for older women needing to supplement the household income. Tourism has become one area in which women can readily find employment.

As tourism employees, women work in a range of occupations: as cleaners, waitresses, bar staff, croupiers, tour guides, receptionists, secretaries, accountants, travel agents, shopkeepers, managers and administrators. Women's choices with regard to tourism employment are circumscribed both by their individual qualifications and experience, and by the social and cultural pressures which apply to women in general and to which women working in the leisure field are particularly subject. Public space remains largely the province of men, especially for purposes of leisure; and to *gezmek*, i.e. to 'be out and about', is overwhelmingly a male pastime which combines socializing with the circulation of information and opportunities to establish useful contacts. Elsewhere I discuss the ways in which the female division of tourism labour reflects cultural boundary concerns and women's role as markers of identity (Scott 1995a). Here, my concern is to explore the heterogeneity of the female workforce and the opportunies offered by tourism employment. Skills, education and experience, economic objectives and constraints, as well as age, marital status and nationality, are all variables which determine both women's demand for particular types of work and what kind of work they are able to get. In the following sections, I briefly examine these characteristics.

Skills, education and experience

Tourism draws heavily on the traditional domestic skills of women (Castelberg-Koulma 1991); but, unsupported by educational or vocational qualifications, or the resources for opening their own businesses, the experience which women have gained from their domestic role tends to translate into 'unskilled' and relatively poorly paid jobs. Cleaning and chamber-maiding is the most readily available work for unqualified women, not least because they face no competition from men for these jobs. The expansion in women's higher education has, however, raised women's expectations. High school and university graduates whose own parents, in many cases, spent their working lives in farming, expect to work in white-collar jobs; and, whereas in the past, such jobs were chiefly restricted to banking or government offices, tourism is increasingly being looked to as a source of white-collar employment.

Several women I spoke to with degrees and high school diplomas had initially applied for public sector/civil service jobs, and had taken up employment in the accountancy and administration departments of large hotels as a result of delays in obtaining their first-choice post. One woman, a trained dental technician, had started her job in the hotel shop after the dental laboratory she had established went out of business. In a few cases, tourism employment remained a second best, but nevertheless a welcome option, given the general lack of opportunities for qualified personnel elsewhere in the economy. Other women, however, were extremely enthusiastic about their job, finding it both busy and rewarding, and commented that were they now to be offered their original first-choice job they would not take it, preferring to stay in hotel employment. A major source of satisfaction was the sense of being *üretken* (productive) – almost all the women in white-collar tourism jobs volunteered the opinion that they were contributing to the wealth of the country by working in the 'locomotive sector' of the economy, and felt that their individual effort made a difference:

'For a long time, I tried to get a job working in a bank – I wanted something a bit dynamic, not working as a government employee drinking coffee all day. . . . People sometimes prefer working in the public sector because, although the pay is about the same, the conditions are better – 42 days' sick leave, pensions . . . if you have a cold, you don't go in to work, whereas I come in even with a cold, and on Saturdays – sometimes in the summer I don't even have time to go to the toilet. People say to me, "Now it's election time, you should try for a public service job, they're taking on lots of people who just sit around with nothing to do." But I don't want a job like that, I prefer to be where I am.'
(High school graduate, personal assistant to general manager in large four-star hotel)

'There is no alternative to tourism on an island such as Cyprus, there are no raw materials, and with the embargo [on Northern Cyprus] export markets are limited. The land is too arid for agriculture. Something is needed which is productive [*verimli*] – at the moment, half the workforce is unproductive [*verimsiz*], in government employment. But you can see the potential for tourism to contribute to the economy in places like Spain. . . . When I first graduated, I really wanted to work in the State Planning Office, since this is the field in which I am qualified and I wanted to use my skills. But here you have the problem that, although the government pays for people to study and get qualifications, the country cannot utilize the skills of all its qualified people. When the hotel [where she had worked for three years] opened, I applied to the accounts department because I had studied accounting at university and because I wanted a 'back-office job' – I don't like to be dealing face to face with people, I like to get on with my own work. Within its limits, the job is OK – it's clean, and people treat you with respect.'

(Masters graduate in economics, working in four-star hotel)

For some other women, choosing a career in tourism has become a route into acquiring vocational and academic qualifications. The state's hotel and tourism school trains young men and women in a variety of the technical tourism skills and qualifies them for middle-ranking work as assistant waiters, bar staff, receptionists and house-keepers.[5] University graduates in tourism are amongst those women who have opened their own business as travel agents in partnership with their husbands. Tourism has, therefore, widened the range of opportunities for women both to gain and make use of vocational training and educational qualifications.

Economic objectives and constraints

Women enter the tourism field with differing economic objectives and constraints. Those who have academic and vocational qualifications seek pay and responsibility commensurate with their skills and educational status; for recent graduates in particular, the work they obtain is a source of prestige both to themselves and their family, and many young women are prepared, with their family's support, to wait for the 'right' job rather than to accept low-status work.

In other cases, women's work, either within their own family's business or as employees, primarily serves household economic strategies, rather than individual social and economic objectives. Most of the women I spoke to who were working as cleaners had been housewives before starting cleaning work, and had taken paid employment either because of a change in family circumstances (such as losing their husband), or to provide an additional source of household income, often to meet a particular item of household expenditure (such as paying for children's university education):

'I have worked at the Dome for eight years, before that I was a housewife. I started working because we needed the money to pay for the children's education – we put all three through university. After I had written my application for a job at the Dome, I spent eight months whilst I waited to be called working at a restaurant – cleaning, washing up, doing general kitchen work. There are 15 cleaners at the Dome, all of them are women. Two of my friends who started at the same time as me have just retired – to get a full pension you have to be at least 55 and have worked for 15 years, although you can retire with less service at 55 and get a proportion of your pension. I wish it were me retiring! But I am only 51. How can anyone work to the age of 55, especially in tourism? I am happy with the pay and conditions, but the work is very hard, especially if we are very busy and I have 18 rooms to clean – I come home from work aching all over.'

(cleaner in large public-sector hotel)

In hotels and guesthouses of all sizes, staff turnover was lowest amongst the cleaners, and in some cases they had remained at the same establishment since it had opened, even when the average length of stay of other employees was only a few months to a year. The average wage was about £100 sterling per month (just above the legal minimum), and whilst a few of the biggest hotels paid £175 sterling, such jobs were not easy to come by, and the waiting lists for them were long. In contrast most of the women working in the white-collar jobs referred to above were earning between £250 and £275 sterling per month.

Age and marital status

Age and marital status are important factors affecting women's economic objectives; likewise, it is mostly younger women who have had the opportunities to gain educational qualifications. In addition, both a woman's domestic commitments outside work and the nature and efficacy of social and cultural constraints on women doing certain types of work tend to vary with age and marital status.

Some tourism jobs – such as cleaning, secretarial and accounts – are day-time jobs with regular hours. Others – including tour guiding, reception, waitressing and bar work – are characterized by irregular and unsocial hours, sometimes through the night. In several large hotels, the hotel shop remains open until midnight during the summer season, and departmental managers are regularly rostered for night shifts as 'duty managers'. For one young woman I spoke to working as assistant general manager of a large hotel, these departures from the 9–5 routine were part of the excitement and attraction of the job, and reinforced in her a sense of competence and self-worth. At the same time, however, she and her husband wanted to have children, and she did not see how she would be able to reconcile the conflicting demands of job and family:

> 'Women doing full-time work have it very difficult. Nobody here really works only their eight hours, and once or twice a week I have to take my turn sleeping over [at the hotel]. This is not popular with my husband, although he has got used to it. But he is looking forward to having children. It would be impossible for me to do my present job part-time, or as a job share. But if I work like I am now, I'd never see my child – and I am concerned about the quality of childcare available. On top of that, you know, women here still do all the cooking and cleaning at home.'
>
> (assistant general manager in large holiday complex)

A single mother working at the same holiday village relied on the flexibility of the management to overcome her childcare problems:

> 'My husband and I are separated. My little boy is 5 years old now, and goes to school, but working and mothering are very difficult. When I get home from work I have to cook and clean, and he sits and watches TV, which I don't like because there is a lot of violence on television. . . . I started working here as a waitress, but the shiftwork made it difficult to get childcare – I don't have any family here who could look after him, they are all in Turkey. A year ago I started working in the hotel shop. The hours are 8am to 4pm, and in the summer I have to work until midnight one night a week. I had a problem in the school holidays, and I brought my little boy in with me every day for weeks. I was worried that I would get into trouble for doing this, but nobody told me off.'
>
> (hotel shopkeeper in large holiday complex)

The practical problems, which women shoulder, with regard to tourism work and domestic commitments, are compounded both by the continuing strength of traditional gender roles, and by the division of labour in the moral economy represented by 'reputation'. Being out at night with strangers, and, in particular, serving them with food and drink, can make a woman the object of gossip and endanger the reputation both of herself and the men of the family. Responsibility for a woman's reputation rests with male kin, and is assumed by the husband on marriage.[6] Younger, unmarried women can sometimes overcome family objections to doing certain types of job, but the objections of a husband, particularly when accompanied by domestic and childcare commitments, are usually harder to resist. According to several hotel managers, women tend to leave jobs as receptionists upon getting married or having children, and very few female tour guides are married. Many travel agencies, on the other hand, are run as husband-and-wife partnerships (six out of a sample of twelve), with the wife supervising the office and taking charge of telephone contacts and ticketing, whilst the husband takes care of outside contacts, visiting tourists and hotels, collecting and delivering tickets, etc. – a case of a division of labour and social space which incorporates traditional gender roles and minimizes the potential for damage to reputation.

'Outsider' status: migrant female workers

Foreign workers may bring skills, knowledge and experience which local workers do not have. Several foreign tour operators employ their own representatives in Northern Cyprus because of their familiarity with the language, culture and requirements of tourists from their own country, and some foreign tour guides are employed by local agencies for the same reasons (especially German speakers, who are in short supply in Northern Cyprus). Tourism's need for foreign language speakers has also provided openings for the daughters of migrants returning from Britain and Australia, as receptionists, hotel telephonists and tour guides. In addition, female migrant workers do those jobs, particularly in the entertainment field, which are socially and culturally unacceptable to Turkish Cypriot women: waitressing in tavernas, working as casino croupiers, or as singers, dancers or night-club hostesses. Such work is usually performed by mainland Turkish women and, increasingly, migrant female workers from former eastern bloc countries.

These migrant workers from Eastern Europe, overwhelmingly Russian and Romanian women, seek work in Northern Cyprus for a number of reasons: to travel and see the world; to escape the conditions of poverty at home; to send remittances back to their family; or to save for some big expense, such as the building of a house. Several of the women have professional qualifications, as doctors, teachers and so on, but are unable to make ends meet on their salary at home. Their association with prostitution has spread to Northern Cyprus from Turkey, where they are known as 'Nata-shas'; and the common use of this name for all Russian and Eastern European women tends to reinforce local people's belief that 'these women are all the same'. The highly sexualized stereotype of the 'Natasha', embodying the exotic, attractive but dangerous outsider, and the absence of family pressure on these women working away from home, frees them from the constraints of reputation to perform those jobs which are not considered 'respectable' for Turkish Cypriot women.[7] At the same time, the stereotype is a burden which the individual women have to bear:

> 'I like it here, and I intend to stay, so that I can pay for my sister's schooling. It's a funny thing, but since Romania became "free" we have to pay for everything – including education. And I am very fond of my sister. I have to watch my money, even though there are more things to spend it on here than in Romania. But sometimes it's difficult living in such a small place. My boss hears even when I have just been to the supermarket. You have to watch your friends – men and women – in case they have a bad reputation. Being Romanian, people judge you all the time. There are too many Romanian girls who come to do dirty things, and men always make assumptions about you. At work I have to be very serious, so as not to give people the wrong idea, and it's hard, because we always used to laugh and joke with the boys at work in Romania. I don't smoke or drink, I haven't had a boyfriend since I have been here, and I don't go to discos.'
>
> (Romanian croupier employed in town centre casino)

These, then, are some of the diverse characteristics and require-ments of the female tourism labour force. In the next sections I examine how the supply of jobs in the tourism sector is structured, and I start with a brief survey of tourism businesses in Girne.

TOURISM BUSINESSES IN GIRNE

According to Ministry of Tourism figures, there are 57 accommoda-tion establishments in the Girne region (i.e. both in town and close to outlying villages), with a combined total of 4,358 beds. Of these establishments, twenty are classified as 'hotels'; ten as 'guest-houses'; and 27 as self-catering 'hotel apartments' (OTP 1993). As part of my research, I conducted interviews with owners, managers and staff at 25 of these establishments, and at twelve of the approximately twenty travel agencies in central Girne.[8]

Although Ministry figures distinguish three types of accommodation, for the purposes of registration and regulation a two-tier system is operated. Establishments with more than ten rooms are regulated by the Ministry of Tourism, and are awarded a star-rating on the basis of their facilities (such as air conditioning, restaurant, swimming pool, etc.). Only the hotels in this category qualify for assistance in the form of incentive credits at subsidised interest rates, tax relief on equipment and furnishings, etc. Guest- and boarding-houses with fewer than ten rooms come under the regulation of the municipality. Like the larger establishments, they pay tax on every tourist they accommodate, which goes towards local services such as refuse collection and water supply, but they receive no financial support and no star classification. Generally speaking, *pansiyon*s are not considered 'proper' tourist establishments – an evaluation which their owners commonly share, since most of their custom comes from 'luggage tourists' and transient migrant workers for whom the main priority is cheapness. The low opinion in which this accommodation sector is held is reinforced by the proliferation of unlicensed premises, which often have very low standards of service and cleanliness (Martin 1993). At the same time, several *pansiyon*s have attempted to upgrade their premises in order to cater to young backpackers from Europe, and Turkish families holidaying on a tight budget.

Later in this chapter, I discuss in some detail differences between the various sectors of accommodation in Girne. Whilst I have retained the Ministry classification for *pansiyon*s (i.e. establishments with fewer than ten rooms), I have divided the remaining hotels in my sample into two groups according to the criterion of ownership structure. This requires some elaboration, particularly since many of the hotels in the sample were in Greek Cypriot and foreign ownership up to 1974. A para-statal organization, created in November 1974, took over the running of the abandoned hotels and leased them to Turkish and Turkish Cypriot managers on a long-term basis. In the past few years, Turkish Cypriots who left property in the south have been allocated points to the equivalent value of the property they left behind, which they have been able to trade in for newly created Turkish Cypriot deeds to houses, land and businesses in the north. Some of the hotels in the sample have been 'bought' in this way, whilst others have been newly built on land acquired with *eşdeğer* (equivalent value) points, or on land which was already in Turkish Cypriot ownership before 1974. Most of the largest hotels, whether acquired with *eşdeğer* points or newly built, are owned by institutions: that is, they are run by the state, by Evkaf (the foundation which administers the property of the mosque), by trade unions, or by private companies, such as Polly Peck, or individuals in partnership with the state. Of the hotels in my sample, I classify such 'institutionally owned' businesses as 'Group I' establishments (see Table 4.1).

In contrast, Group II hotels (see Table 4.2), are in individual or family ownership, or run as a partnership between two or three individuals. Whilst they are considerably larger than *pansiyon*s ('Group III' businesses), they are, on the whole, much smaller than Group I hotels.

The smallest businesses are those in Group III (see Table 4.3). In only one case (no. 3) were premises purpose-built for accommodating tourists; in all the other cases the businesses were run in converted houses, which were either rented, or bought with *eşdeğer* points.

Group I and II business have several characteristics in common: they come under the regulation of the Ministry of Tourism, are eligible for various types of government support, and cater for European and Turkish tourists – that is, they work with travel agents who have links to the Turkish and European markets, and either the owner, or some of the staff, speak English or German. Group III businesses, in contrast, cater for a less affluent market, and generally rely for publicity on word of mouth rather than on formal relationships with travel agencies. On the other hand, Group II and Group III establishments can be seen as representative of a range of

Table 4.1 Group I: 'institutionally owned' accommodation by number of employees and size

Hotel	no. of beds	Total employees	Female employees
A	305	120	n.a.
B	392	163	50
C	152	85	24
D	126	55	20

Source: Tourism Planning Office Statistics 1992 and personal interviews
Note: Includes hotels and self-catering establishments, and core number of permanent employees. Hotels A, B and D include a casino on the premises: the number of casino staff is not shown.
n.a. – data not available

Table 4.2   Group II: 'family businesses' – privately owned hotels by number of employees and size

Hotel	no. of beds	Total employees	Female employees
E	166	60	n.a.
F	44	2	0
G	28	5	2
H	32	9	5
J	36	14	6
K	40	2	0
L	24	4	1
M	48	6	2
N	44	5	1
O	100	4	1

Source: Tourism Planning Office Statistics 1992 and personal interviews
Note: Includes hotel and self-catering accommodation and core number of permanent staff, with exception of hotel E (number employed in high season – in low season a skeleton staff of 13 was employed); and hotels F and K (staffed mainly on family labour – only numbers of non-family staff shown). Hotel E includes a casino on the premises; the number of casino staff is not shown.
n.a. – data not available

family-run businesses: both tend to employ considerably fewer staff per bed than Group I hotels; the proceeds of the business provide income for an individual or household, rather than a company or

Table 4.3   Group III: 'family businesses' – guesthouses and boarding houses (fewer than ten rooms) by number of employees

Pansiyon	Total employees	Female employees
1	3	1
2	1	1
3	3	1
4	0	0
5	0	0
6	0	0
7	1	1
8	1	1
9	3	1
10	1	0
11	1	1

Source: Personal interviews
Note: Establishments 4, 5 and 6 use only family labour.

institution, and the businesses dispose of correspondingly smaller resources.

For the purposes of this discussion, I contrast the institutionally owned businesses in Group I with the 'family businesses' in Groups II and III. As will become clear, however, the input of *family labour* in these businesses is variable, and can often be strikingly low. Only four hotels in Group II (F, H, K and M) relied heavily on the labour of family members (husband, wife and grown-up children); with two exceptions, the remaining hotels in the group were owned and run by married men, employing entirely non-family labour. The input of family labour was slightly higher in Group III: in three cases, all the work was done by members of the family; in another three cases (nos 2, 8 and 11), family labour was supplemented by the employment of a cleaner; and in the remaining five cases, no family labour was involved. In all Group III businesses, and all but three of Group II (E, H and J), women were employed only as cleaners; female family labour also tended to be restricted to cleaning and cooking, and rarely included reception, bar, restaurant or management work. In Group I hotels, in contrast, women feature in a wide range of occupations, including cleaning, restaurant and bar service, reception, administration and management. In the next sections I examine the reasons for this pattern, and I start by looking at women's participation in family businesses.

WOMEN IN FAMILY BUSINESSES

Several factors may favour a strong role for women in the family business sector. Taking paying guests enables women to combine domestic work with earning an income whilst remaining in the home. As Bouquet (1982) has pointed out, this permits a partial commoditization of women's domestic labour which can be pursued as a strategy of household pluriactivity. In the case of farmhouse bed and breakfasts in Devon studied by Bouquet, and in the Spanish seaside town studied by Hermans, women took responsibility for tourism business whilst men continued their occupations in agriculture and fishing. This division of labour is encouraged by a 'natural' slow (i.e. 'organic', cf. Cohen 1972) growth in tourism: '[Women] could start on a very small scale, their husbands doing the "real" work in fishery and agriculture' (Hermans 1983: 21). According to Hermans, women were able to maintain control of their business once tourism had superseded farming and fishing as an economic activity because the enterprise was viewed as an extension of the household, women's traditional sphere. The tradition of partible inheritance, with daughters inheriting the family house whilst sons inherited the fishing boat, further consolidated their position. Reynoso y Valle and de Regt also found that female employment was greatest in those businesses controlled by women: 'Female managers are more likely to hire women for a wider range of hotel positions' (Reynoso y Valle and de Regt 1979: 131).

Why, then, do women appear to be marginal to this sector in Girne? I suggest three reasons: first, the spatial arrangements for accommodating guests; secondly, the process of tourism development in Northern Cyprus; and thirdly, the pattern of household pluriactivity.

Premises

Guests are not accommodated in the family home. In all but two cases, the family dwelling was some distance from the tourist accommodation, frequently in another neighbourhood or village. In the other two cases (both small *pansiyon*s in Group III) there was no connecting access between guest and family accommodation, and the household lived in a separate building or storey on the same plot of land. Maintaining this spatial separation not only avoids conflict over 'domestic' and 'guest' use of space which is a common problem of taking paying guests into the home (Bouquet 1987; Ireland 1993), but it also avoids possible gossip which would be damaging to the sexual reputation of both the women and the men of the family, and which would almost certainly accompany the opening of the family home to overnight stays by strangers, particularly men. It is significant that in one of the two *pansiyon*s mentioned above, where family residence adjoined guest accommodation, the wife and daughter did not participate directly in the running of the business, although the wife had her own job as a school cleaner. In the case of the other *pansiyon*, which was run by a single man with his elderly parents, the age of the mother precluded the possibility of gossip and she was frequently to be found in the reception area, chatting to guests. This spatial arrangement means that the business cannot be run as a spin-off from women's domestic work, and prevents women establishing the sort of niche described by Bouquet and Hermans, even though the practice of partible inheritance in Northern Cyprus means that women frequently own the premises in which the business is being carried out.

The process of tourism development in North Cyprus

According to Hermans, the slow development and natural growth of tourism in Cambrils enabled women to build up a business gradually from small beginnings and consolidate their position by the time tourism had become established. Tourism in Northern Cyprus has not shown the type of 'slow and steady' growth which is a feature of 'organic' tourism development (Cohen 1972), but has been characterized by contradictory trends. After 1974, Northern Cyprus's tourism could be said to have been 'supply led' in terms of available hotel stock, but with few skilled staff and virtually no tourists. The problem of international transport communications which has continued to dog Northern Cyprus's tourism has meant that there has not been a steadily increasing stream of independent travellers from Europe to enable a small business using largely domestic labour and space to develop from scratch. Most businesses have to rely on organized group travel, with travel agents packaging and selling Northern Cyprus as a destination and simplifying the travel arrangements from Europe. This involves even relatively small businesses in a variety of formal relationships, and in a greater outlay in order to bring accommodation up to a standard expected by package tourists. It is men who form the social and business contacts, queue in government offices, apply for bank loans and so on – a division of tasks which the women I spoke to appeared to accept without question.[9] At the same time, the budget market from Turkey, which for at least the first ten to fifteen years consisted largely of luggage tourists and male migrant workers, has contributed to the generally poor reputation locally of *pansiyons*, particularly in the capital, Lefkoşa (Nicosia), which would deter most women from opening a business in this sector.

Far from being a subsidiary activity, tourism has been designated the 'leading economic sector', its high profile enhanced by the relative lack of more lucrative alternatives. In Northern Cyprus the features of tourism development most favourable to the type of women's small-scale involvement described by Hermans and Bouquet appear to be largely absent.

Household pluriactivity

In the model of pluriactivity proposed by Bouquet and Hermans, non-productive labour and resources (in the sense that they are non-commoditized or produced for use) are brought into the realm of exchange values in order to increase household resources. This is not the pattern of pluriactivity which emerges from the sample of Group II and III businesses in Girne. It can be seen from Table 4.4 that in three cases wives were involved in some other form of business or employment outside the hotel/*pansiyon*; in seven cases, wives were working with their husband and sometimes

Table 4.4 Pluriactivity in Groups II and III

Hotel	Wife's occupation	Husband's other business activities
Group II		
E	n.a.	TR
F	in hotel	TR
G	housewife	
H	in hotel	NTR
J		
K	in hotel	NTR
L	own business	NTR
M	in hotel	
N	n.a.	NTR
O	n.a.	TR
Group III		
1		
2		NTR
3	own business	
4	in *pansiyon*	NTR
5	employed	other employment
6	housewife	other employment
7	housewife	
8	in *pansiyon*/restaurant	TR
9	housewife	TR
10	housewife	NTR
11	in *pansiyon*/restaurant	TR

Source: personal interviews
Note:
TR: tourism-related activity
NTR: non-tourism-related activity
The owners of establishments J, 1 and 2 were not married.
n.a. – data not available (but in all cases wife was not actively involved in hotel business)

with other members of the family in the hotel/*pansiyon*; and in eight cases the wives do not appear to be economically active. On the other hand, reference to the 'other business activities' column shows that roughly three-quarters of the businesses in the sample (i.e. fifteen out of twenty-one) had other sources of household income, and it is probable that the proportion is higher if unregistered business activities are taken into account. It became apparent in the course of interviews that the creation of additional sources of income was largely due to the diverse activities of the husband, who at the same time maintained an active and usually leading role in running the accommodation business.

Group II hotels are well-resourced compared to Group III businesses, and employ a higher proportion of non-family staff (see Tables 4.2 and 4.3). The non-tourism related activities pursued in this group included citrus cultivation, animal husbandry, estate agency, construction and import/export trade, and in most cases these had pre-dated entry into the hotel business. Some of these households had access to inherited wealth which they were able to use for investment in premises. The other tourism-related activities pursued by hotels E and F were fairly small-scale, consisting of shares in a high street restaurant and a shop and travel agency; hotel O's operations were much larger, and included car hire, money change, a casino and travel agency. Husbands combined the hotel business with other commitments, and were able to do this because their activities were largely entrepreneurial, giving them flexibility and the resources to hire workers where family labour was not used.

Group III *pansiyon*s have fewer resources available for investment. In two cases, additional income was gained from 'other employment' rather than self-employment, and in two other cases (2 and 4) income from other business activities was sporadic. Only three guesthouses had been purpose-built (1, 2 and 3); in the other cases, the availability of unutilized space had prompted entry into the accommodation business.[10] In five cases (5, 6, 8, 10, 11) accommodating guests was a sideline to the main business (of restaurant, patisserie and other employment).

Women's roles were marginal to the business in all but four cases: business 1, whose owner was an expatriate woman with Turkish Cypriot citizenship; business 4, which provided the main source of income for the family and also suffered the greatest resource constraints of the sample;[11] and 8 and 11, in which husband and wife worked as a partnership within a diversified tourism business in which the high-quality restaurant, the main responsibility of the wife, played an important part. The role of the wife in 3 and 9 had declined as businesses had become more successful and husbands had followed a strategy of diversification within their particular business niche (increasing the number of rooms and expanding into snack bars and car hire). Such diversification is usually the product of partnerships between male kin and business associates, rather than using a wife's domestic labour.[12]

Compared with the availability of other resources, the use of non-commoditized domestic labour is relatively unimportant to household pluriactivity strategies in Groups II and III. Women's most important contribution is usually as a channel for the transmission of inherited wealth and property. New resources tend to be generated by the business activities of men which depend on male kin networks, social contacts, access to information and so on, whereas Turkish Cypriot women have only recently become economically active outside the home, and there is no established tradition of independent female entrepreneurship. Women were most visible as active managers in hotels H and M, where their husbands were involved in non-tourism related businesses which frequently took them away from the hotel and the wives' participation represented substantial savings on the cost of hiring skilled personnel.[13] Unskilled labour, on the other hand, is relatively cheap and where family businesses have the resources to hire domestic labour, there is no 'need' for a wife to double her workload by doing housework in the hotel as well as at home.

WOMEN'S PARTICIPATION IN INSTITUTIONALLY OWNED BUSINESSES

Institutionally owned hotels differ from family businesses not only in terms of their size and the numbers employed, but also organizationally. Group I hotels are characterized by the 'bureaucratization' of hospitality (Shamir 1978), with professional managers and a hierarchical authority structure, and opportunities for promotion and career development. Staff were organized into departments, each dealing with a separate aspect of the business: typically these consisted of front-office/reception; back-office (administration and accountancy); service (dining room and bar); housekeeping; and technical/maintenance. Each had a departmental manager reporting to the general manager or the assistant manager. In addition, one hotel with computerized reservation and accounting systems had a computer manager, and two had a food and beverages manager.

Quality and professionalism of service are important in these top-of-the-range hotels, both for the satisfaction of the customer and the image and reputation of the hotel. Managers emphasized the importance of recruiting and retaining skilled staff: standards in pay and conditions of employment tended to be considerably better than those in most family hotels, and included an extra month's salary per year, various allowances, and index-linking every two months to keep salaries in pace with the high inflation rate. Management attempted to promote an ethos of discipline and high standards amongst the staff and apply criteria of merit in recruitment and promotion.

According to a study of a new tourism development of large, luxury hotels in Mexico close to an existing village containing small, family hotels, women formed a significantly lower proportion of the employees in the new businesses than they did in the older hotels in the village. Furthermore, 'Women are more likely to be owners or managers of the older hotels and to work as chambermaids, secretaries, and, in one case, waitresses in the new' (Reynoso y Valle and de Regt 1979: 131). In the sample of hotels in Girne, the situation is more or less reversed, although men still do predominate in Group I, both as managers and in terms of the total number of employees (see Tables 4.1, 4.2 and 4.3 on pp. 74 and 75).

The proportion of female staff in the hotels in Group I varied from about one-third to nearly one-half of the total, although the majority of female employees was concentrated in the housekeeping department, which in all cases was composed entirely of women, whilst staff in the service departments (bar and restaurant) were nearly all men. Two hotels had a couple of women working as restaurant waitresses or barwomen, but reported little demand from women for this sort of work. Opposition to women working in the service department came from family and from male waiters rather than from management, who maintained that they choose and promote staff on the principle of 'the best person for the job'. One young woman who had worked in restaurant service said that she had experienced hostility from her male colleagues, because, they said, women could not do the job and were more suited to cleaning. Their attitude, combined with the problems of finding childcare when she was working an evening shift, had led her to leave the service department and move over to the hotel shop. A high proportion of women worked in hotel casinos, both as croupiers and waitresses; almost without exception these were not Turkish Cypriot women, but Rumanian, Turkish, or British.

Women typically formed 30–50 per cent of employees in other departments (with the exception of technical/maintenance departments which were all-male). Secretarial, administrative and accountancy posts are attractive to women, being white-collar work with a regular 9–5 day, which enables them to be at home in the evening. Women in these positions were usually high school graduates, although some had accountancy qualifications and one had a Masters degree in economics. Working at reception was also popular, particularly for women with language skills. Although reception desks are staffed 24 hours per day with three eight-hour shifts, rotas usually ensured that women work the day shift, whilst all-male shifts were rostered for the night time. Hotel shops were also staffed by women.

Whilst male employees significantly outnumbered female in Group I (see Table 4.1), findings from the sample suggest a different interpretation from that of progressive exclusion of women with the greater 'professionalization' of large hotels. The multiplicity of functions within a large organization creates opportunities for women to work outside the traditionally male-dominated service and technical departments, for example in back-office jobs and hotel shops. In addition, the size of the workforce permits greater flexibility to roster women for day shifts in those jobs, such as reception work, which need 24-hour-a-day cover.

The position of women was also helped by the adoption of an ethos of 'rational management', which was often stressed by managers as an important attribute in a modern hotel. Their emphasis on modern, rational management methods can be seen in part as a response to Northern Cyprus's isolation outside the mainstream, and the desire to be judged in terms of professional international standards as an effort to compensate for that isolation. Gender was said not to be an issue in employment; rather, male and female managers and most of the women employees interviewed considered the division of labour in the hotel where they worked to be the outcome of cultural preferences in society at large, not management decisions; and many managers considered that they were ahead of society in their employment policies.

The question remains, whether women tend to be concentrated in jobs which pay less than those done by men. It proved difficult to establish points of comparison between, for example, the typical wage for a cleaner and a waiter, as individual wages varied according to personal service increments and monthly bonuses. On the whole, the basic pay for waiters and cleaners was roughly the same at the equivalent of about £150 sterling per month, although waiters tended to receive a greater bonus from the 10 per cent service charge paid by customers and shared amongst employees in all departments. The greatest source of discrepancy lay in the low numbers of women at departmental manager rank and above, which placed a ceiling on an individual woman's earning potential. In three out of the four Group I hotels, the only female manager was the head of the housekeeping department. In the fourth hotel, out of a total of eight there were two female managers, one of whom was the assistant general manager; in addition, the food and beverage supervisor was a woman.

CONCLUSION

Women play an important role in tourism in Northern Cyprus, but control of tourism remains largely in the hands of men. From this somewhat bald statement I should like to draw out some more specific conclusions which relate both to the case of Northern Cyprus and to tourism gender issues more generally.

With regard, first of all, to the question of tourism's power to transform gender roles, tourism development in Northern Cyprus does not appear to be tending towards any such transformation, but rather to be incorporating and extending existing values and relationships; and in fact I would argue that this is a common pattern. Other case studies cited above have shown that women's control of small-sector tourism enterprises is based on existing gender roles and the division of household labour. Family businesses in Girne also reinforce the existing division of labour: one in which men take responsibility for businesses and deal with outside contacts, a pattern which, as Reynoso y Valle and de Regt predict, also results in fewer women being hired as employees. At the same time, the demand from women for white-collar employment, previously limited to the urban middle and upper classes, has increased dramatically with the expansion in women's education, and the employment opportunities offered by large hotels have gone some way towards meeting this demand. It is in this sector that shifts in gender roles and relationships seem most likely to occur. Whilst resource constraints and the nature of the tourism market limit the pay and prospects of female employees in family businesses, large-scale establishments, with their access to greater resources, can offer a wider range of work opportunities to women, and greater flexibility in working conditions.

Women's entry to the labour market is a relatively recent phenomenon, but they are starting to break into management positions in Group I hotels. Changes in attitudes to women's employment in large hotels have been gradual, occurring over a period of years rather than overnight. One woman, now the housekeeping supervisor at a prestigious hotel, said that her family had objected when she started working in hotels 20 years earlier and had insisted that her older brother collect her from work every day. Today it is particular jobs in tourism rather than hotel employment *per se* which might raise family objections – in particular, waitressing and bar work. But the presence of a migrant female workforce has so far allowed most of these jobs to be filled from 'outside the community', pre-empting any challenge that these new jobs might present to ideas about women expressed in the code of reputation. Indeed the stereotype of the shameless woman represented by 'Natasha' appears to have reinforced women's symbolic function as boundary markers and the role of reputation in delineating the local community (Scott 1995a). What is striking is the persistence, in the face of tourism development, of pre-existing gender roles and relationships, albeit manifested in new contexts and new forms.

This brings me to my second point: the phenomenon, occasionally noted in the literature, but not much commented on, of the degree of self-exploitation by women in the family accommodation sector of their own domestic labour. Whatever the benefits to women of running their own accommodation business, it also entails an increase in domestic work, long hours, and a decline in social interaction with neighbours and kin, an aspect of the business which women complained of in studies by Kousis (1989) and Hermans (1983). The women I spoke to could well understand why a woman who owned a guesthouse would not want to increase the amount of domestic drudgery in her life, especially given the availability of cheap migrant labour from Turkey to do the work. The question remains why more women, as owners or co-owners of premises, are not themselves more active as employers and managers; and I suggest that it is gendered access to social space and management of social and business relationships which provides an explanation for this.

Castelberg-Koulma argues, from the evidence of women's agro-tourism co-operatives in Greece, that women's business activities gave them increased confidence to move into public spaces and business relationships outside the community which had previously been the province of men (Castelberg-Koulma 1991). In Northern Cyprus the problem may be simply that there has not been enough of the right kind of tourism to stimulate this kind of movement amongst women. However, the cases discussed above suggest that the situation is actually more diverse. On the one hand, women's success as travel agents has so far not transformed gendered use of space and business and information networks: women's duties keep them in the office, whilst men combine responsibility for outside contacts with the traditional male activity of *gezmek*. On the other hand, in large hotels, women are starting to become visible in jobs and departments which were previously closed to them. Recognizing that these variations exist, and coming to some understanding of the mechanisms for change, requires an analysis which sets the gendered division of labour in the context of the status of the work (white-collar, skilled, unskilled, prestigious and so on), the nature of the space in which it occurs (for example village, urban, home, guesthouse, hotel, etc.), and the cultural meanings attached to the gendered use of these spaces, both for work and for leisure.

A further point is that individual decisions to work or not to work in the tourism field also take place in the context of collective ideas about tourism and development, which may take the form of 'public opinion' in general or officially promoted ideologies in particular. Attitudes in Northern Cyprus appear to bear out the findings of a recent study which found that views held about tourism cut across gender lines, even though men and women do not benefit equally from tourism development (Harvey *et al.* 1995). In Northern Cyprus, this unanimity of view, I suggest, arises at least in part from the belief in tourism's importance as part of the national struggle to achieve recognition and prosperity on a par with the Greek Cypriot south.

As the officially designated 'locomotive sector' it falls to tourism to modernize the economy and replace the traditional dependence on agriculture. This goal of 'modernization' is one which is widely shared by Turkish Cypriot women as well as men. In terms of the type of tourism development envisaged, sustainable alternatives to mass tourism (such as village tourism, agro-tourism) are, so far, not on the agenda; rather, both women and men expressed the opinion that Northern Cyprus must first of all 'catch up' and enter the mainstream. In the large hotels, this attitude can work in women's favour. The self-conscious ethos of 'modern' and 'rational' management, in the context of the boycotts on Northern Cyprus, has the symbolic function of asserting a place for Turkish Cypriot tourism in the international mainstream from which it is excluded. It also benefits women by encouraging meritocratic rather than gender criteria in recruitment and promotion.

Finally, the diversity evident in the choices and chances of women in Turkish Cypriot tourism highlights the need for an explanatory framework which takes in the differences between women as well as their commonalities as women, and the interplay between gender and other factors to produce particular outcomes. This is to echo Henderson's call for an approach which seeks explanations in pluralisms rather than dualisms, adopts 'multiple theories giving a range of explanations for varied circumstances', and sets the context of gender by '[locating] gendered actors within social landscapes' (Swain 1995: 255). In Northern Cyprus ethnicity, class, wealth, education and the moral evaluations to which women are subject intersect with gender divisions of labour and space, public ideologies of nationalism and development, and the composition of the tourist market, to make up the 'circumstances and relationships that shape choices of gendered behaviour' (ibid.: 255).

NOTES

1 Research was for a Ph.D. degree and was funded by the Economic and Social Research Council. Fieldwork was carried out from mid-1992 to December 1993.
2 I give the Turkish names of places in Northern Cyprus, some of which were used by Turkish Cypriots before 1974, whilst others are new Turkish names created since the division of Cyprus. When a place name is first mentioned, the name most familiar to English speakers follows in brackets. On the issue of place names in Northern Cyprus, see King and Ladbury (1988).
3 For example, out of 100 billion Turkish lira credit which Turkey granted to Northern Cyprus in 1993 for sectoral development, tourism received 60 billion Turkish lira, more than any other economic sector, whilst agriculture was allocated only 15 billion Turkish lira (*Yeniduzen* 23.2.93).
4 Many of these are abandoned Greek Cypriot properties which the

Ministry of Tourism has made available on long-term lease (usually up to 35 years) to foreign nationals willing to restore them in 'traditional' style and materials.

5 Between 1974 and 1992, there were 497 graduates from the hotel and tourism school, of whom 88, or roughly 18 per cent, were female (OTP 1993).

6 At the same time, men and women tend to evaluate reputation according to different criteria and in different social contexts. For a discussion of gender differences in the evaluation of honour and shame, see Wikan (1984) and Scott (1995b).

7 For a fuller discussion of reputation in relation to female tourism employment and the role of migrant women workers, see Scott (1995a).

8 Numbers fluctuate as businesses open and close: for example, two additional travel agencies had opened in Girne by the end of 1993. The collection of tourism statistics by the Ministry lags behind actual events such as the opening and closing of travel agencies, guesthouses and boarding houses, and Ministry figures currently under-represent the number of *pansiyon*s in the Girne region. My sample included eleven *pansiyon*s in central Girne alone.

9 According to one informant, husband and wife partnerships are often registered only in the husband's name because it is he who deals with official bureaucracy, a situation which she accepted because 'women can't queue in offices and deal with that side of things'.

10 Unutilized space means an additional house (e.g. an inherited house) rather than space within a house.

11 Two generations, consisting of elderly parents, married couple, and husband's sister, ran this *pansiyon* together without employing outside labour. Other income (from videoing wedding and circumcision celebrations in the summer) was sporadic; in addition, the family, which had moved to Girne from the south of Cyprus in 1974, had not yet obtained deeds to the property they had been allocated and had no collateral to raise loans for the business.

12 This can also include the male kin of a wife.

13 Even so, a male manager or '*sorumlu*' was often employed to deputize for the husband. My sample suggested a difference in this respect between the practices of Turkish Cypriot families (where wives were more visible in managerial roles) and families from Turkey, but, owing to time constraints, this was not a point I was able to follow up during fieldwork.

BIBLIOGRAPHY

Armstrong, K. (1977) 'Women, Tourism and Politics', *Anthropological Quarterly* 50, 3: 135–46.

Berner, U. (1992) *Das Vergessene Volk* (The Forgotten People), Pfaffenweiler: Centaurus.

Boissevain, J. and Inglott, P. S. (1979) 'Tourism in Malta', in E. de Kadt (ed.) *Tourism: Passport to Development?*, Oxford: Oxford University Press.

Bouquet, M. (1982) 'Production and Reproduction of Family Farms in South-West England', *Sociologia Ruralis* 22, 3/4: 227–44.

—— (1984) 'Women's Work in Rural South-West England', in N. Long (ed.) *Family and Work in Rural Society*, London: Tavistock.

—— (1987) 'Bed, Breakfast and Evening Meal: Commensality in the Nineteenth and Twentieth Century Household in Hartland', in M. Bouquet and P. Winter (eds) *Who From their Labours Rest? Conflict and Practice in Rural Tourism*, Aldershot: Avebury Press.

Bryden, J. (1973) *Tourism and Development: A Case Study of the Caribbean*, Cambridge: Cambridge University Press.

Castelberg-Koulma, M. (1991) 'Greek Women and Tourism: Women's Co-operatives as an Alternative Form of Organization', in N. Redclift and M. T. Sinclair (eds) *Working Women: International Perspectives on Labour and Gender Ideology*, London: Routledge.

Cohen, E. (1972) 'Towards a Sociology of International Tourism', *Sociological Research* 39, 1: 164–82.

Çağın, H. (1990) 'Structural Changes in Tourism', in *Proceedings of a Conference on Structural Changes in the Economy of Northern Cyprus, 3–4 December 1990*, Gazi Mağusa: University of the Eastern Mediterranean.

Garcia-Ramon, M. D., Canoves, G. and Valdovinos, N. (1995) 'Farm Tourism, Gender and the Environment in Spain', *Annals of Tourism Research* 22, 2: 267–82.

Harvey, M. J., Hunt, J. and Harris, C. C. (1995) 'Gender and Community Tourism Dependence Level', *Annals of Tourism Research* 22, 2: 349–66.

Hermans, D. (1983) 'Spanish Women in Business: The Case of Cambrils', *Etnologia Europea* XIII, 1.

Ioannides, D. (1992) 'Tourism Development Agents: The Cypriot Resort Cycle', *Annals of Tourism Research* 19, 4: 711–31.

Ireland, M. (1993) 'Gender and Class Relations in Tourism Employment', *Annals of Tourism Research* 20: 666–84.

King, R. and Ladbury, S. (1988) 'Settlement Renaming in Turkish Cyprus', *Geography* 73, 4: 363–7.

Kousis, M. (1989) 'Tourism and the Family in a Rural Cretan Community', *Annals of Tourism Research* 16: 318–32.

Ladbury, S. (1979) 'Turkish Cypriots in London: Economy, Society, Culture and Change', unpublished Ph.D. thesis, University of London, School of Oriental and African Studies.

—— and King, R. (1982) 'The Cultural Construction of Political Reality: Greek and Turkish Cyprus Since 1974', *Anthropological Quarterly* 55, 1: 1–16.

Lockhart, D. and Ashton, S. (1990) 'Tourism to Northern Cyprus', *Geography* 75, 2: 163–7.

Loizos, P. (1981) *The Heart Grown Bitter: A Chronicle of Cypriot War Refugees*, Cambridge: Cambridge University Press.

Martin, J. (1993) 'The History and Development of Tourism', in C. H.

Dodd (ed.) *Political, Social and Economic Development of Northern Cyprus*, Huntingdon: Eothen Press.

Morvaridi, B. (1993) 'Agriculture and the Environment', in C. H. Dodd (ed.) *Political, Social and Economic Development of Northern Cyprus*, Huntingdon: Eothen Press.

OECD (1988) *Tourism Policy and International Tourism in OECD Member Countries*, Paris: OECD.

OTP (1993) *Tourism Statistics 1992*, Lefkoşa (Nicosia): Office of Tourism Planning (in Turkish and English).

Purcell, H. D. (1969) *Cyprus*, London: Ernest Benn.

Repena-Osolnik, M. (1983) 'The Role of Farm Women in Rural Pluriactivity: Experience from Yugoslavia', *Sociologia Ruralis* 23, 1: 89–94.

Reynoso y Valle, A. and de Regt, J. P. (1979) 'Growing Pains: Planned Tourism Development in Ixtapa-Zihuatenejo', in E. de Kadt (ed.) *Tourism: Passport to Development?*, Oxford: Oxford University Press.

Samarasuriya, S. (1982) *Who Needs Tourism? Employment for Women in the Holiday Industry of Sudugama, Sri Lanka*, Colombo/Leiden: Research Project Women and Development.

Scott, J. (1995a) 'Sexual and National Boundaries in Tourism', *Annals of Tourism Research* 22, 2: 385–403.

—— (1995b) 'Identity, Visibility and Legitimacy in Turkish Cypriot Tourism Development', unpublished Ph.D. thesis, University of Kent at Canterbury.

Shamir, B. (1978) 'Between Bureaucracy and Hospitality: Some Organizational Characteristics of Hotels', *Journal of Management Studies* 15, 3: 285–307.

Smaoui, A. (1979) 'Tourism and Employment in Tunisia', in E. de Kadt (ed.) *Tourism: Passport to Development?*, Oxford: Oxford University Press.

Swain, M. (1995) 'Gender in Tourism', *Annals of Tourism Research* 22, 2: 247–66.

SPO (1981–1992) *First, Second and Third Five Year Development Plans*, Lefkoşa (Nicosia): State Planning Organization (in Turkish).

Wikan, U. (1984) 'Shame and Honour: A Contestable Pair', *Man* 19: 635–52.

Chapter 5

Gender and tourism development in Balinese villages

Veronica H. Long and Sara L. Kindon

INTRODUCTION

The field of tourism studies is relatively young and, as such, is still establishing its basic tenets. In addition, gender analysis within tourism studies is even younger and the integration of the two bodies of tourism and gender research is, in fact, almost never seen (Richter, 1994). However there are some recent exceptions to this void (Kinnaird and Hall, 1994; Swain, 1995). The material presented in this chapter examines four vignettes of Balinese tourism development from a gender perspective. We trust that such an analysis will contribute to the growing understanding of the interaction between tourism and gender occurring in various types and at various scales of development.

The chapter opens with overviews of tourism development and the indigenous and political systems of gender relations within which the tourism development is occurring in Bali. We then draw upon four vignettes to illustrate the interaction between varying types of tourism development and the gendered impacts or modifications at different scales in each place. Finally, we examine in more depth the common processes underlying the four vignettes and provide some reflections on how women, in particular, have affected and been affected by the tourism development.

TOURISM DEVELOPMENT AND GENDER IN BALINESE SOCIETY

Tourism development in Bali

Tourists have been coming to Bali to see the culture and physical beauty of its environment since the 1920s. Some of these early visitors formed a colony of foreign artists and anthropologists who focused their attention on the interior of the island, in the vicinity of the village of Ubud (Universitas Udayana and Francillon, 1975; Picard, 1990; Sutton, 1991) (Figure 5.1). These resident expatriates, experts in a number of cultural fields, nurtured the arts in the area and helped spread the word regarding the rich cultural attractiveness of the island (Picard, 1990; Sutton, 1991).

In 1969, with the construction of the Ngurah Rai International Airport in the south of the island (Figure 5.1), mass tourism began and the number of tourists increased dramatically. Most of these tourists stay in the southern region of Badung and Gianyar as it is there that 80 per cent of all tourist accommodations, and 98 per cent of all star hotels may be found (Dibnah, 1992) (see Figure 5.1). Australians make up a great deal of the recreational market segment; they come on charter vacation packages and tend to stay in and around the cities of Kuta and Sanur (Mabbett, 1987). In addition, the island caters for visitors from Europe, North America and Japan who represent the majority of the cultural market segment. These tourists explore more parts of the island, but tend to concentrate their visit in the Ubud area.

When Indonesia started focusing on socio-economic development in the late 1960s, the tourism industry in Bali was chosen for its potential to attract investment and international attention. A tourism master plan for Bali, (SCETO, 1971) was written by a consortium of French consultants, and sponsored by The United Nations Development Program (UNDP) and the International Bank for Reconstruction and Development (IBRD). This plan proposed that tourism development be concentrated in enclaves in the south with excursion routes into the interior of the island. The approach was designed to protect the Balinese culture from potentially harmful tourism impacts (SCETO 1971; Rodenberg 1980) and maintain its attraction as an exotic, mystical unspoilt paradise.

Many resident Balinese responded to the influx of young, low-budget, 'drifter' tourists in the 1960s, opening small-scale businesses, restaurants, 'homestays' (bed and breakfast inns), souvenir shops, and art manufacturing enterprises (Noronha, 1976). By the late 1980s, these businesses formed a large and thriving informal sector in Bali's economy (Wahnschafft, 1982). In 1988, the Balinese provincial government changed its concentrated approach to tourism development planning and adopted a policy designed to diffuse economic benefits throughout the island. This approach allowed

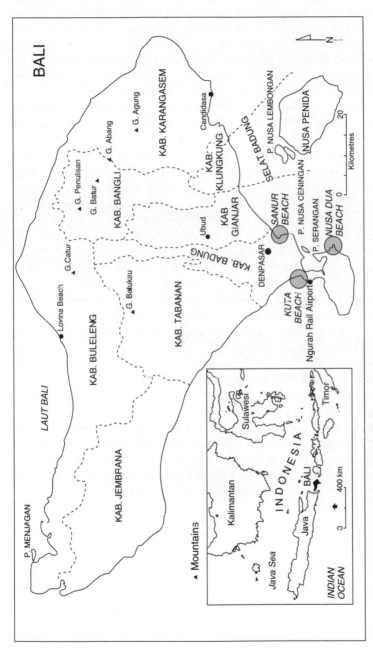

Figure 5.1 Principal tourism areas in Bali
Source: Wall, 1993

for a more equitable distribution of tourism development opportunities. It also represented a more realistic approach to the spontaneous development already taking place as a result of weak development control mechanisms (Dibnah, 1992).

Today, it is indisputable that, for Bali, tourism development is one of the most dynamic forces shaping its economy (Gertler and Tjatera 1990). The majority of investment in Bali is occurring in the accommodation and service sectors, and agriculture and other manufacturing industries are also increasing to support the service sector.

The impact of tourism on Balinese culture and society, however, is less clear cut and has long been a source of concern and debate (Universitas Udayana and Francillon 1975; Noronha 1976; Picard 1990). Some writers such as Lansing (1974), McTaggart (1980), Mabbett (1987), and McKean (1989) suggest that tourism is not having a negative impact on Balinese society, while others, like Francillon (1990), describe the phenomenon as a 'tragedy'. Picard (1993) asserts that tourism is not an external agent of change in Bali, that it is transforming Balinese society, and is being transformed by Balinese society from within. He also suggests that it should be seen in the broader context of the colonization and 'Indonesiazation' of Bali by the Javanese-dominated central Government of Indonesia (GOI) in Jakarta.

Tourism development is a formidable force affecting Bali in many ways, but its impacts on gender in Balinese society have received little attention. Balinese society is well known for its unique ability to adapt to external social forces (Universitas Udayana and Francillon, 1975; Picard, 1990; Wall, 1990; Geriya, 1991). It seems to have internalized tourism development making it conform to Balinese interpretation. This interpretation puts tourism and its impacts into categories which are sensible for Balinese society, thus reducing the stress of adapting to tourism development.

Indigenous and political systems of gender relations in Balinese society

According to Balinese Hinduism and *adat* (customary practice), women and men are born to be free and should have equal rights and obligations (Wiratmadja, 1991). However, perceptions of women and men, and their roles and relations in society, are shaped by religious and ideological symbols, attitudes and values (Miller

and Branson, 1984) as well as by the GOI's political ideology and
practice (Suryakusuma, 1991; Hermawati and Kindon, 1993).

For example as shown in Tables 5.1 and 5.2, men are regarded as
the primary members of their families who act as their head (*kepala
keluarga*), public representative, manager and decision maker. They
are considered to be rational, active, intelligent and strong. Women,
on the other hand, are viewed as secondary to, less intelligent, and
less confident than men. They are considered to be passive and
emotional, and are valued as care-givers and implementors of
decisions who are responsible for their families' private needs
(Ruddick, 1986; Hermawati and Kindon, 1993; Kindon, 1993b).

The Balinese socio-cultural system is, therefore, one in which
women and men are espoused to be equal, but different. This
ideological difference results in women's and men's performance
of distinct gender roles within a hierarchical relationship where men

Table 5.1 Women's qualities as described by a group of Balinese
villagers

Women's positive qualities	Women's negative qualities
Play a strong role in *adat*	Shy/reluctant to attend meetings
Close to family, responsible and help husband to increase family income	Sometimes lazy, do not work, just ask husbands for money[1]
Easier to teach and involve in development than men because keen to learn new skills, start hobbies and be productive	Have low education and awareness which limits the use of new technology/information to improve their situation
Efficient users of time	Lack tenacity if they fail at something
Willing and effective motivators and supporters of husbands	Not strong enough for heavy or night work
Better coordinators than men because patient, flexible and willing to disseminate information	Too emotional to make rational decisions
Thorough, patient, diligent and neat	
Skillful traders and money managers	

Source: Kindon (1993: 100)
Note: [1] This assessment was expressed by male participants only.

e 5.2 Men's qualities as described by a group of Balinese villagers

en's positive qualities	Men's negative qualities
Play strong role in *gotong royong* (mutual self-help) and village unity	Like gambling, cock fights and visiting prostitutes
Physically strong and work hard	Do not support or allow women's participation in development
Greater earning capacity than women[1]	Many are lazy and do not fulfill their role as primary income earner[2]
Organizers and planners	Do not respect women leaders
Keen to learn	Low education limits use of new technology/information to improve their situation
More educated/informed than women	Poor disseminators of information
Creative and imaginative	

Source: Kindon (1993: 101)
Notes: [1] This assessment depends on wages and perceptions of 'work'.
[2] This assessment was expressed by female participants only.

are the organizers and women the organized (Miller and Branson, 1984).

Within the Balinese Hindu patrilineal kinship system, for example, women and men do not have equal rights. Women do not usually inherit land upon marriage or parental death (although this is changing with increasing education and urbanization), women have no rights to their children or marriage property if they divorce, and women are not allowed to be polygamous (Kindon, 1993a; Ariani, 1990). Men, on the other hand, inherit land, keep their children and property upon divorce and may have more than one wife.

In addition, the Balinese Hindu caste system serves to inhibit women's equality and social mobility by preserving the hierarchical status of men in marriage and society. For example, an unfavourable marriage is one between a woman of higher caste and a man of lower caste. In this case, the hierarchy of gender relations is unbalanced and the woman is cast out by her family. This type of caste restriction upon marriage only applies to women because:

> While women do not actually transmit any of their own caste standing to children, they either transmit paternal blood lines undiluted, or they negatively affect paternal lineage by giving

birth to children who are a notch or two below pure offspring in the same lineage.

(Ruddick, 1986: 95)

As such, men hold a critical and higher position than women in family and community life (Koencaraninggrat, 1970) and women are defined in relationship to men whom they are expected to respect and honour as the master of the family and household (Ariani and Kindon, 1994). Consequently, sons are valued more highly than daughters and receive preferential treatment with respect to access to resources and education (Hermawati and Kindon, 1993).

This indigenous ideological positioning of women within a hierarchical relationship with men is also reinforced by GOI political ideology and practice. Women are encouraged to follow the Five Duties of Women (*Panca Dharma Wanita*) which are defined as follows (see Suryakusuma, 1991: 52):

1 Loyal companion to the husband.
2 Manager of the household.
3 Educator and guider of children.
4 Supplementary wage earner for the family.
5 Useful member of the community.

Women in Development (WID) approaches (Kindon, 1993b; Moser, 1989), act as a strategy of control over women through the glorification of motherhood (Suryakusuma, 1991). WID policies generally aimed at enhancing the role and status of women in development projects have been noted for being Euro-centric and economically biased. They place women in the contradictory position of having to balance multiple roles as reproductive care-givers, economic producers and community managers (Ariani and Effendie, 1989; Moser, 1989; Wiasti, 1989; Arjani and Wiasti, 1991; Hermawati and Kindon, 1993; Norris, 1994). For women in Bali, the tension associated with these roles is particularly marked because of their additional responsibilities as the preparers and presenters of daily and ceremonial religious offerings.

In addition, at nearly all levels of decision-making (government and indigenous *adat* systems), men occupy leadership positions and control the decision-making process. While, in theory, women are eligible to attend meetings with men, they often must await invitations from male decision-makers who have the power to decide if the meeting will concern 'women's issues' or not (Kindon, 1993b).

Consequently, women are not generally invited to meetings about such matters as village water supply systems because they are of a technical nature, despite the fact that women remain largely responsible for the collection of their families' water supplies (Kindon, 1993b; Noerhajati et al., 1993).

With regard to income generation and work, women have traditionally been economically autonomous in Bali's informal sector working in trade and small business to provide for their families' needs (Miller and Branson, 1984; Mabbett, 1987; Kindon, 1993b). In recent years, however, their autonomy has been overlooked in favour of WID approaches which seek to incorporate women into the formal economy (Norris, 1994). Alternatively, women's economic autonomy has been seen as a threat (Norris, 1994) and has been undermined through the re-establishment of relations of ruling (Smith, 1987) through a reintrenchment of male dominance (Miller and Branson, 1984).

The nature of women's productive activities are influenced by the modes of their reproductive responsibilities (Norris, 1994). Women's participation in the formal economy as well as their spatial mobility and location of work are thus largely defined by indigenous and political ideologies associated with their gender and marital status.

The resultant gender division of labour means that women and men tend to operate in distinct social and economic spheres with women being under greater pressure to balance their multiple roles (Kindon, 1993a). As more women enter tourism, gender ideologies and the balancing of roles and relations are extended into, and/or renegotiated within, these new areas of economic activity. The four vignettes below examine some of the ways in which tourism and gender interact to change gender relations and the impacts of tourism development.

FOUR VIGNETTES OF GENDER AND TOURISM DEVELOPMENT IN BALI

To examine the interaction of gender and tourism development at a local level in Bali, we have selected four vignettes gathered from recent research by us and our colleagues associated with the Bali Sustainable Development Project (BSDP). BSDP was a five-year project administered by the University Consortium on the Environment and the Indonesian Environmental Management and Development Center. The project was managed by a team of environmental studies personnel from The University of Waterloo in Ontario, Canada and Gajah Mada University in Java, Indonesia, in association with Udayana University in Bali, Indonesia. BSDP sought to devise a strategy for sustainable development to inform the Balinese provincial planning process. A major focus of the BSDP investigations was on the role of gender in Balinese society. Because of this focus, a great deal of attention was paid by field researchers to the conditions and processes of Balinese life.

First, we explore 'homestay' development in Desa Peliatan, near Ubud, from research conducted in 1991 by Veronica Long and Geoff Wall (Long and Wall, 1995). Second, the development of the gold and silver handicraft industry is examined in Desa Celuk in Gianyar. The information is based on work by academics from the Women's Study Centre at Udayana University (Ariani *et al.*, 1992 in Kindon, 1993a). Third, we detail the recreational tourism in Desa Jungut Batu on Nusa Lembongan from work conducted by Long in 1993 and 1994 (Long, 1995), and fourth, Joanne Norris's (1994) work on informal and formal tourism development in Desa Kedewatan near Ubud is analysed. Figure 5.2 shows the locations of the vignettes presented.

Vignette 1: family homestays

The Ubud region is noted as the centre of cultural arts in Bali (Santosa, 1980; Manuaba *et al.*, 1989; Mantra, 1991) and is comprised of several scenic river valleys with beautiful panoramas of terraced rice fields. Desa Peliatan is heavily integrated with the socio-economic activities of the village of Ubud due to its geographic location and complementary tourist attractions. A *banjar*, or neighbourhood, in Desa Peliatan was chosen for study because, along with its focus on cultural arts and performances, it was experiencing rapid development of homestay accommodation in what was considered 'a smaller and quieter version of Ubud' (Dalton, 1990).

In the *banjar* during 1991, Long and Wall noted 25 homestays, three restaurants, six stores with some souvenirs, and six foodstalls (*warungs*) operated by members of the 200 resident families. In particular, the 'homestays' or *losmen* were characterized by their small size, family-ownership and operation, and low prices (Santosa, 1980). They were typical of the accommodation provided

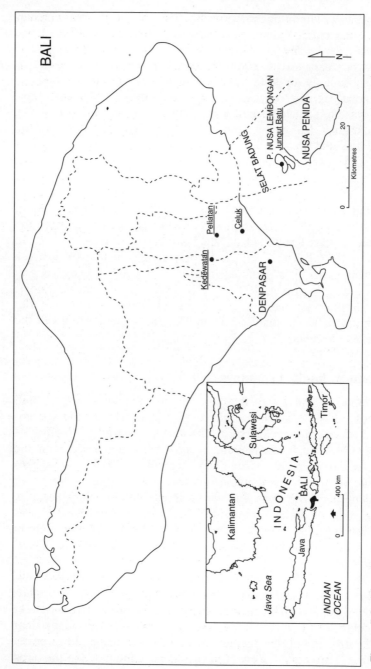

Figure 5.2 Vignette locations
Source: adapted from Wall, 1993

by Balinese residents elsewhere on the island, offering rooms with two single beds and bathroom, breakfast and desired views of traditional housing compounds and family life. The widespread development of such homestays not only represented a supply of inexpensive accommodations to serve the low-budget market, but also demonstrated the tourists' demand for interaction with the Balinese.

All 25 of the homestays in the *banjar* were surveyed. All but one of the homestays were owned by the resident families and were co-managed by the male and female members of the household compound. Half of them were staffed by family members, seven by hired labour, and three by a combination of family and hired labour. Most of the day-to-day work was carried out by the female head of the household compound and this included such tasks as cooking breakfast, cleaning the rooms, providing hot tea all day, doing laundry, and shopping for food.

As most of the male heads of household held outside employment, the bulk of the management duties were left to the female head of household. They would cook and serve breakfasts, with tea and coffee in the morning, clean the rooms, and negotiate room prices with newcomers. In addition, they often took visitors to the market with them and included them in *banjar* ceremonies which included lending them traditional clothing and helping them to dress.

As the survey was done quickly and only to document development, no in-depth study of homestay accounting could be done. Although the researchers' observations were supported by an earlier study by Udayana University (Manuaba *et al.*, 1989), which showed very little accounting done in family businesses, revenue, expenditures, and profits were not clear.

The development of homestays was taking place quite rapidly, with eleven of the 25 surveyed having been constructed in the previous eleven months. This was despite the fact that only twelve of those families had any previous experience in tourism-related business, and two others admitted to learning about the business as they went along. In the future, sixteen of those families intended to build one or more extra rooms and two wanted to provide hot water.

The rapid development of these successful enterprises also created tension and rivalry among *banjar* families. Several homestay operators indicated that they didn't like the low revenue caused by bartering and competition. One resident confided that he was worried that black magic would be used like in Ubud among rival businesses (Long and Wall, 1995).

However, when conflicts arose, a new organization was formed among the *banjar* members involved in tourism, to make decisions about the future management of their community's development. As with traditional *banjar* membership, however, the organization's members were restricted to male heads of household compounds. One female homestay operator who wanted to attend a meeting was told not to by her husband (Tani, personal communication, August 1991). Thus, women as the main providers of daily labour and management in all the homestays surveyed did not have a voice in the critical processes of conflict resolution or decision-making for future community tourism development.

Vignette 2: silver and gold craft shops

Desa Celuk is a major centre of silver and gold production, particularly for the tourist and export markets. It grew in popularity with tourists because of its location on one of the original 'excursion routes' designed to help 'tourists discover the real Bali, its way of life and cultures' (SCETO, 1971). It is a stop-off point for many organized bus tours from Kuta and Sanur and in the last twenty years the number of shops built along the main road has doubled (Suradiya, 1994). These shops have created new jobs and resulted in a 'true cottage industry with almost every family here working at home' (Santosa, 1985: 60). In addition, they have replaced productive rice fields (Wall and Long, 1993) and the need for agricultural labour.

Ariani *et al.*, (in Kindon, 1993a) chose a *dusun* (governmentally designated hamlet) in Desa Celuk as a study area, specifically to investigate whether gender relations, the household division of labour and/or the ownership and control over material property were changing as women and men moved from occupations in farming to silver- and goldsmithing. They used in-depth interviews with members of a sample of ten household compounds using the 'snowballing' method. Life histories were also collected for certain representative households.

Table 5.3 shows the management arrangements in the household businesses. Of note is the fact that women felt their participation as co- or single managers improved their status as they gained recognition from men for their business skills. Equal numbers of women

Table 5.3 Silver and gold household business management arrang_
ments

Management arrangements	% of households interviewed
Joint management by husband and wife	40
Husband manages, wife assists	30
Wife manages alone	20
Wife manages, husband assists	5
Husband manages alone	5

Source: Ariani et al., 1993

and men were employed in the ten household businesses. Most
employees lived outside the village and were unmarried.

In addition to managing household businesses, women tended to
maintain their reproductive roles of care-givers and domestic managers (*Ibu Rumah Tanga*). Thus, while women worked fewer hours
per month in the silver and gold handicraft industry as both employers and employees than men, when combined with their other tasks,
the number of hours worked by women was actually higher (Table
5.4).

In terms of the management of household income resulting from
work in the silver and gold handicraft industry, husbands and wives
most frequently manage the income together, or women have sole
management responsibility. However, if income expenditure is
examined, then major purchases are decided upon by men and are
written under the husband's or married son's names. Women remain
in charge of purchases for daily needs, but their control and ownership of material goods has not increased with their increased
contributions to household income. This continues to undermine
women's personal economic security in the case of such future
events as divorce.

Table 5.4 Hours worked per month by activity, status, and gender

Activity	Income generation silver		gold		Housework		Religious		Social		Total	
Status[1]	a	b	a	b	a	b	a	b	a	b	a	b
Wife (hrs)	166	91	0	150	76	221	35	28	15	18	202	508
Husband	178	216	83	155	4	56	29	11	9	21	303	459

Source: Taken from: Ariani et al., (1993: 34)
Note: [1] Status is signified by 'a' (Employer) and 'b' (Employee).

Vignette 3: day cruises and surfer bungalows

Desa Jungut Batu is one of two villages on the island of Nusa Lembongan, 22 km off the south-east shore of Bali. Most of the population was engaged in seaweed farming, but other activities included boat transport, dryland farming, fishing, small business, and tourism activities.

Long used participant observation and interviews in order to investigate the social impacts of tourism in the village (Long, 1995). Since the early 1970s, low-budget travellers have been attracted to the world-class surfing and the slow pace of the island. Eleven bungalows/*losmen* and two to four restaurants (depending on the high/low season) had been built to accommodate these tourists who came mainly to surf. Wealthier tourists had been attracted to the island on day excursions offered by charter yachts, surfing and diving charter groups, and Bali Hai Cruises, a 300-passenger cruise ship. These tourists mainly focused on water-based activities, such as snorkelling, and had little interaction with the village. The main exception was tourists on one of the three daily Bali Hai tours of the village.

Many villagers supplemented their income from seaweed farming with tourism work. For example, Bali Hai employed eight villagers on regular salaries and eleven through contracts associated with the village tours. Of the employees, only one salaried employee and five contract workers were female. However, in the art shops associated with the village tours the majority of employees and managers are women (20 out of 26 workers). On the other hand, in the eleven bungalows/*losmen* and five restaurants, more men than women worked as managers (Table 5.5), while approximately equal numbers worked as hired staff as cleaners, cooks, waitering staff, or some combination thereof. These hired staff were mostly between

Table 5.5   Gender and status of bungalows/*losmen* managers

Gender and status	% of bungalows/losmen
Resident male	46
Resident female	27
Resident male and female	9
Hired male	18
Hired female	0

Source: Long, 1995

the ages of 15 and 22 and all were unmarried. Four of the homestays were owned jointly by husbands and wives, the rest were owned by men.

Elsewhere, all 32 registered captains that ferried passengers and cargo between Sanur beach and Desa Jungut Batu everyday were male. Furthermore, all guides (accommodation and snorkelling or transport) on the island were also male.

Vignette 4: exclusive hotels and family shops

Desa Kedewatan lies on the Ayung River ravine 5 kilometres from Ubud. Tourism developed in the form of hotels, homestays, art and souvenir shops since 1980. Desa Kedewatan differed from Ubud as most of its accommodations were either moderately priced ($30–$50 US) or exclusive ($100–$700 US). Land along the scenic Ayung River was either sold or contracted out and villagers who had previously been stuck with steep, less arable land suddenly became the *nouveaux riches*.

Norris's work involved participant observation and interviews with 73 tourism workers between the ages of 16 and 45 and employed in a variety of tourism occupations as shown in Table 5.6. The village has had a stable population with most villagers continuing to be employed in agriculture (Norris, 1994). However, increasing numbers of young people were finishing high school and seeking tourism training diplomas to gain employment in the village's growing number of hotels, art shops and dance groups.

Norris reported that many respondents told her that the increased wealth was increasing the amount of gambling and extra-marital affairs by men in the village.

Most art shops were still small, family-operated and located on or near the male household head's family compound. Many of the shops were operated by a husband and wife team, unless the husband was

Table 5.6 Tourism employment distribution by gender

	Hotel	Homestay	Restaurant	Art shop	Souvenir shop	Other	Total
Male	20	2	4	5	3	1[1]	35
Female	24	1	2	5	6		39
Total	44	3	6	10	9	1	73

Source: Norris, 1994
Note: [1] tour guide

employed elsewhere in which case the wife alone managed the business. Some of these women had worked in one of the hotels prior to marriage, but had left to work in the family shop where it was easier to balance domestic and community responsibilities with paid work.

In restaurants, approximately equal numbers of unmarried women and men worked as cooks, or waitering staff. In contrast, work in the exclusive hotels was noticeably gender segregated. Positions of security guards, drivers, grounds keepers and maintenance staff were occupied by men, while women (mostly unmarried) worked in the housekeeping, restaurant, or accounting sections. All of these jobs paid substantially better than the other jobs in Desa Kedewatan, but were held mainly by outsiders who had higher skill-levels than local residents.

UNDERLYING PROCESSES OF GENDER-RELATED IMPACTS OF TOURISM DEVELOPMENT

The four vignettes described above provide sketches of the gender-related impacts associated with various types and scales of tourism development. The main impacts are summarized in Table 5.7.

From Table 5.7, it would seem that while tourism development at the village level in Bali is clearly providing new avenues of employment for women and men, the development itself is causing little change in their more fundamental relationships with each other. In fact, it could be argued that the types of tourism development occurring in these four vignettes is actually reinforcing existing systems of gender perceptions, roles and relations which determine that women continue to take responsibility for reproductive activities regardless of other work, and that men continue to have greater access to positions of authority and decision-making.

We suggest that the existing indigenous and political systems of gender ideology, combined with the type and scale of tourism development occurring in Bali, serve to reinforce the hierarchies assumed to exist between women and men, and between informal and formal developments. In summary, the structures of gender and tourism development tend, upon interaction, to be self-reinforcing and perpetuating.

By way of illustration of the above point, let us consider the influence of each in turn.

Table 5.7   Summary table of gender-related impacts from four vignettes

	Gender-related impacts
Family homestays	• increased work for women in reproductive and informal sector activities • maintenance of male-dominated access to and control over decision-making and community management • generally, the existing household gender division of labour (GDOL) and hierarchical gender relations are reinforced
Silver and gold craft shops	• increased work for women in addition to reproductive activities • greater freedom to gain formal work for unmarried women • increase in working women's status in community • maintenance of existing GDOL and hierarchical gender relations • little improvement in women's economic security
Day cruises and surfer bungalows	• GDOL is reinforced according to job type • men have access to and participate in formal salaried work (higher status work) and women undertake more informal work (lower status work) • greater freedom to work for unmarried women
Exclusive hotels and family shops	• informal and formal sectors reinforce GDOL • increased work for women in addition to reproductive activities • greater freedom to work for unmarried women

Indigenous and political gender ideologies

As we detailed in the first section of this chapter, the indigenous and political gender ideologies in Bali, and Indonesia in general, are highly influential upon the perceptions, roles and relations considered appropriate for women and men. Most of the ideologies are based upon a tacit assumption of biological determinism, i.e., that the biological characteristics of women and men determine their social characteristics. There is optimism about increasing women's role in the tourism workforce, but even this optimism is coloured with a gender bias as can be seen in the following statement, 'A beneficial factor is the possibility that parts (of the tourism industry) need the feminine characteristics of female employees more than simply manpower' (Universitas Gadjah Mada, 1993).

Although tourism employment is being considered as a way to integrate women into roles with higher profiles in Indonesian society (Universitas Gadjah Mada, 1993), in the new opportunities provided by tourism development, jobs tend to be divided along socially appropriate lines. For example, guiding is determined to be more appropriate work for men to do because it is not socially acceptable for an unmarried woman to be alone with foreign men. Moreover, outside or physical work such as employment as groundstaff (Kedewatan), and/or involvement in boating (Jungut Batu) is seen as an extension of men's work in agriculture and more in keeping with their perceived greater physical strength. An example of the prevailing Indonesian perspective is reflected in the following presentation based on Sadli (1992: 103–5):

Women are particularly well suited for work in cultural tourism because:

1 Women are socialized to be sensitive to the needs of others.
2 Women are reputed to be verbally better than men at language acquisition so they can learn foreign language easier.
3 Women are normally caring and good at routine jobs.
4 Women are more attractive than men.

In addition, these gender ideologies influence where women and men can work throughout their life cycles. Men are generally free to work wherever they need to and many migrate to tourism developments and live away from home. As a result, they have greater access to both formal and informal employment sectors within tourism. For women, they too are able to migrate to work until they get married. Then they are expected to stay closer to their family to be able to carry out their reproductive duties as wives and mothers. In Indonesia married women have a lower rate of participation in the labour force than single women (Hugo et al., 1990). Young unmarried women in Celuk, Jungut Batu and Kedewatan all expressed that they would have to leave their jobs upon marriage and look for more informal work, closer to home. Typically, this kind of work would be running a warung or souvenir shop which would allow them flexibility to look after children and attend to community responsibilities.

Alternatively, women in the vignettes often, upon marriage, set up businesses with their husbands (Peliatan, Celuk, Jungut Batu and Kedewatan). Commonly, restaurants, homestays and *losmen* provide a socially acceptable way for women to earn extra income through the extension of their other gender roles to care for tourists in the informal sector. Such work in homestays demands that women work longer hours to balance all their tasks, yet this extra work often goes unnoticed because it is so similar to their other responsibilities.

Although there are many benefits through direct employment in a small-scale enterprise, as in Bali, it is often the case that businesses such as bed and breakfast inns increase the workload for household women (Fairbairn-Dunlop, 1994; Long and Wall, 1995; Smith, 1994). In Ireland, Armstrong (1978) shows most of the work goes to women but none of the political power goes to them. Richter (1994) points out that in general terms, 'women have the majority of the jobs at the base of the tourism employment hierarchy and men have almost all of the jobs at the middle and top.' In Bali, men occupy most formal positions of power and thus control decision-making at all levels of Balinese society (Hyma and Kindon, 1992).

Men too tend to assume work that follows the acceptable division of labour. As such they undertake more formal work in hotels or as guides and drivers. Table 5.8 shows how men far out-number women in the employment of guides. They continue to be managers of property and information (Peliatan, Celuk) and with their higher status in society, have access to decision-making forums and authority related to household and community affairs. In none of the results of the four case study vignettes did women gain any increased control.

This situation is reflected elsewhere in Indonesia as in a study by Gadjah Mada University (1993) which reports 'society still doubts women's ability to decide policy in the tourism industry,' (1993: 149). This study analysed the role of women in tourism in five provinces and found that women generally have a moderate amount of access to and participation in tourism though their control of the industry is weak. Table 5.9 shows some of the results of the study.

The Balinese situation is not only seen throughout Indonesia, but has also been reported elsewhere by other researchers. Many studies have shown that prevailing gender perceptions result in the types of tourism employment that men and women have (Fairbairn-Dunlop, 1994; Lim, 1992; Norris, 1994), and that male/female divisions in

Table 5.8 Development of licensed guides in Bali, 1984–1991

Language specialization	1984 M	F	T	1985 M	F	T	1986 M	F	T	1987 M	F	T	1988 M	F	T	1989 M	F	T	1990/1991 M	F	T
English	174	3	177	185	3	188	220	2	222	261	5	266	297	6	303	495	14	509	657	26	683
French	43	1	44	43	1	44	48	1	49	57	1	58	45	2	47	48	4	52	55	5	60
Italian	38		38	38		38	39		39	47		47	30		30	63	1	64	84	2	86
German	20	1	21	20	4	24	20		20	30	2	32	25	3	28	29	4	33	37	6	43
Japanese	113	8	121	119	8	127	133	9	142	207	21	228	234	25	259	249	39	288	348	55	403
Spanish	20		20	20		20	20		20	20		20	22		22	16	1	17	22	1	23
Dutch	15	1	16	15	1	16	14		14	18		18	11	1	12	16	1	17	18	2	20
Mandarin	1	1	2	3	1	4	4	2	6	6	2	8	13		13	22	2	24	23	3	26
Arabic	1		1	1		1	1		1	1		1	1		1	4		4	4		4
Swedish	1		1	1		1	1		1	2		2	0		0	0		0	0		0
Korean	1		1	1		1	1		1	1		1	0		0	0		0	2		2
Total:	427	15	442	446	18	464	501	14	515	650	31	681	678	37	716	942	66	1008	1250	100	1350

Source: Tourism Office, Bali, 1991
Note: M = Male, F = Female, T = Total

Table 5.9 Profile of the role of women in tourism in five Indonesian provinces

| Province | | Role (mean % of women in sample) | | |
		Participation	Access	Control/power
North Sumatera	Resource[1]	31.07	34.40	28.07
	Benefit[2]	42.92	35.14	26.81
West Sumatera	Resource	41.88	41.52	31.42
	Benefit	52.89	51.39	43.64
Yogyakarta	Resource	39.90	35.04	30.75
	Benefit	50.82	45.90	32.45
West Nusa	Resource	29.52	26.13	27.14
Tengarra	Benefit	32.26	31.35	29.28
South Sulawesi	Resource	36.83	35.44	28.35
	Benefit	33.92	31.48	25.21

Source: Universitas Gadjah Mada, 1993
Notes: [1] Resource includes: capital, training, marketing and employment
[2] Benefit includes: income, status and information

formal employment are mirrored in the informal areas of employment (Chant, 1993).

One of the major factors influencing women's role in the tourism industry in Bali is a lack of formal education. The general level of education for women in Indonesia is rising but rural women have less that urban women (Thorbecke and van der Pluijm, 1993) and close to one-third of the female urban workforce had no education (Hugo et al., 1990). Women are traditionally involved in textile, basketry, crafts, singing and dancing, but need more access to higher education in order to expand their involvement in tourism (Soebadio, 1992).

Type and scale of tourism development

With increasing tourism development of varying types and scales, women and men have greater opportunities for employment and improved status in society. In most general terms, scale includes concepts of formal or informal types of tourism development. Rodenburg (1980: 179) defines scale as follows: '(1) relative size and capitalization, i.e. physical plant of an enterprise, and its correlate; (2) relative bureaucratization, i.e. degree of industrial organization.' Thus 'small-scale' usually includes informal, and large-scale involves formal tourism enterprises. Type and scale of tourism development are important because they affect employment

opportunities, large-scale generally having less local income distribution than small-scale development (Rodenburg, 1980; Wall, 1993;
Norris, 1994). Table 5.10 demonstrates some of the characteristics
of tourism entrepreneurship in Bali. With growing urbanization and
education in Bali more young people are entering occupations in the
tourist industry. For women, however, the type and scale of the
tourist development influences their access to work.

As we mentioned above, women are often subject to more social
restrictions than men, which affect their social and physical mobility.
Clearly, greater opportunities exist for women in informal types of
small-scale tourism development. Several studies have shown that
women are the main workers in the bed and breakfast industry
(Stringer, 1991; Norris, 1994; Long and Wall, 1995). It is here that
women have the greatest amount of flexibility in their management of
time and gain most acceptance from their families and communities.

Examples from Peliatan, Celuk and Kedewatan suggest that
women are likely to move from work in formal and/or large-scale
to informal and/or small-scale tourism development throughout their
life cycle. Men are less likely to follow this pattern. In addition, it
appears that the more formal and large the type and scale of
development, the more rigid the gender segregation of labour
becomes. There are a greater number of political and social controls in effect from GOI legislation involved with the formal sector
of tourism employment. One example is legislation banning women
from night work to ensure the normal functioning of reproduction
(Norris, 1994). Others address assumptions about women's and
men's abilities for certain types of work (Sadli, 1992; Universitas
Gadjah Mada, 1993).

Table 5.10   Local and foreign entrepreneurship in Bali

			Origin of owner (%)		
Scale of enterprise	number	Local village	Greater Bali	Indonesian foreign	Nature of ownership
Large	5	0	0	100	Corporate
Medium	111	33.3	16.7	50	Corporate/Individual
Small:					
homestay	195[a]	66.7	28.5	4.8	Individual
restaurant	NA[b]	66.7	33.3	0	Individual
souvenir shop	NA[b]	66.7	33.3	0	Individual

Source: Rodenburg, (1980: 191)
Notes: [a] Gross underestimate – figure includes 'homestays' from four areas
          [b] figures not available

Large-scale tourism generally involves employment in hotels, travel and tour agencies, and large and/or urban restaurants. Wall (1993) compared five-star hotels with guest houses, considering their related visitor characteristics and the ways in which they interacted with the economic, cultural and environmental factors of Bali. Accordingly, the five-star hotels had large amounts of formal employment.

It is not clear how formal tourism employee positions are divided between males and females. While one study reported that males outnumber females in front desk jobs, (Hassall and Associates *et al.*, 1992), another found them to be relatively equal (Cukier and Wall, 1995). Another in-depth investigation by Norris (1994) of employment opportunities and constraints in the Balinese village of Kedewatan, found that more opportunities existed for males than females in hotel industry employment.

It is possible to see how increasing amounts of education and urbanization may affect the participation of women in the tourism industry and then affect broader social change. Tourism may precipitate social change, filtering into relatively private spaces as homestays open families to intimate exposure to outsiders (Wall, 1993). In rural Greece, functions relating to the world outside the home were once the male domain but now that rural women's co-operatives that work with tourism have been established, this barrier is beginning to disappear (Castelberg-Koulma, 1991). In Bali, families regularly include tourists in *banjar* ceremonies and women who operate homestays often allowed guests to accompany them while shopping at the local market (Long and Wall, 1995).

CONCLUDING REMARKS

With tourism representing one of the largest sectors in international and national trade, it is essential that we reformulate our focus to identify associated societal change and what it means for women and men.

(Kinnaird *et al.* 1994: 27)

This chapter is an attempt to explore gender-related impacts of tourism development in Bali and to contribute to studies of social change. Four vignettes of village tourism development in Bali were presented in order to demonstrate the various types of situations which exist. Many issues were not included, such as prostitution which is often linked to tourism in south-east Asia (Thanh-Dam, 1983; Lee, 1991; Hall, 1994a) or the creation of gendered areas in the villages (Hall, 1994b). Common themes were seen which were related to type and scale of tourism development and explained in terms of indigenous and political gender ideologies. It was found that when gender ideologies and tourism type and scale interact the strongest reinforcement of socially determined and acceptable divisions of labour occurs with formal and large-scale development. This, in turn, reinforces certain types of access and control over work and income for women.

Can we assume therefore, that Bali's spontaneous small-scale development is more beneficial for women than its more centralized and planned developments? Certainly, women are actively pursuing new avenues of work and increasing their status in society, but their participation in informal and small-scale tourism developments masks the continuing inequities of access to decision-making and more formal authority that are based in Balinese ideology and practice. Rather than transforming cultural traditions (of which gender ideology is one) as many writers have feared, it would seem that tourism development is interacting with systems of gender ideology to strengthen and reinforce the status quo.

Women and men live 'according to their own cultural interpretations of their changing worlds,' (Ong, 1988, as cited by Norris, 1994). The experiences of these men and women will vary by their race, class, and gender. We do not consider these women to be victims and in general believe it is their place, not ours, to subjectively evaluate their situations. It is possible that the higher levels of education and participation in the formal areas of tourism may result in some form of emancipation for women. In this case, those that espouse emancipation of women at the same time as cultural preservation in Bali via small-scale tourism development are faced with a quandary. This chapter has shown that because of enduring traditions and political ideology thus far, there has not been a great deal of change in gender relations in Bali.

ACKNOWLEDGEMENTS

The authors would like to acknowledge the support of the Bali Sustainable Development Project and their colleagues there. The support from Geoff Wall and assistance from Alex Keuper is also very much appreciated.

REFERENCES

Ariani, G. (1990). *Akses Wanita Perkerja Terhadap Harta Benda*. Denpasar, Indonesia: Facultas Hukum, Universitas Udayana.

Ariani, G., M. Effendie. (1989). *Kembang Rampai Wanita Bali*. Denpasar, Indonesia: Kelompok Studi Wanita, Universitas Udayana.

Ariani, G. and S. Kindon. (1994). 'Women, Gender and Sustainable Development in Bali, Indonesia.' in *Bali: Balancing Economy, Environment and Culture*, eds B. Mitchell and S. Martapo. Waterloo: University of Waterloo Press.

Ariani, I. G. A. A., N. L. Arjani, N. M. Wiasati, O. Parwata and A. A. Sukranatha. (1993). 'The Impacts of Tourism upon the Status and Role of Women in Gold and Silver Handicraft Production in Desa Celuk, Kabupaten, Gianyar.' in *Bali Sustainable Development Project: Gender and Development Training Workshop, June 22–23 1992*. University Consortium on the Environment Publication Series Research Paper no. 48. Waterloo, Ontario: University Consortium on the Environment.

Arjani, L. and M. Wiasti, Peranan Wanita Bali Ditinjau Dari Perspecktif Budaya. (1991). Paper prepared for the Bali Sustainable Development Project Denpasar, Indonesia: Universitas Udayana.

Armstrong, K. (1978). 'Rural Scottish Women: Politics without Power.' *Ethnos* 43: 51–72.

Castelberg-Koulma, M. (1991). 'Greek women and tourism: women's cooperatives as an alternative form of organization.' in *Working Women: International Perspectives on Labour and Gender Ideology*, eds N. Redclift and M. T. Sinclair. New York: Routledge.

Chant, S. (1993). 'Working women in Boracay.' *Tourism in Focus* 17: 8–9.

Cukier, J. and G. Wall (1995). 'Tourism Employment in Bali: A Gender Analysis.' *Tourism Economics* 1 (4): 389–401.

Dalton, B. (1990). *Bali Handbook*. Chico, California: Moon Publications.

Dibnah, S. (1992). *An Assessment of Spatial Arrangement Plans for Tourist Areas in Bali*. University Consortium on the Environment Publication Series Research Paper no. 39. Waterloo, Ontario: University Consortium on the Environment.

Fairbairn-Dunlop, P. (1994). 'Gender, Culture and Tourism Development in Western Samoa.' in *Tourism: A Gender Analysis*, eds V. Kinnaird and D. Hall. Chichester, England: John Wiley Sons & Ltd.

Francillon, G. (1990). 'The Dilemma of Tourism in Bali.' in *Sustainable Development and Environmental Management of Small Islands*, eds W. Beller, P. d'Ayala and P. Hein. Paris: UNESCO and Parthenon Publishing Group.

Geriya, W. (1991). 'Culture and Sustainable Development in Bali.' Doctoral dissertation. Denpasar, Bali: Faculty of Letters, University of Udayana.

Gertler, L. and W. Tjatera. (1990). 'Regional Development.' in *Bali Sustainable Development Project: Report on the Second Workshop: Environment and Development in Bali*. University Consortium on the Environment Publication Series Research Report no. 2. Waterloo, Ontario: University Consortium on the Environment.

Hall, C. M. (1994a). 'The Politics of Heritage Tourism: Place, Power and the Representation of Values in the Urban Tourism Context.' in *Quality Management in Urban Tourism: Balancing Business and Environment*, ed. P. E. Murphy. University of Victoria, Victoria Canada, 1994, November 10. Victoria, British Columbia: University of Victoria.

—— (1994b). 'Gender and Economic Interests in Tourism Prostitution: the Nature, Development and Implications of Sex-tourism in Southeast Asia.' in *Tourism: A Gender Analysis*, eds V. Kinnaird and D. Hall. Chichester, England: John Wiley & Sons Ltd.

Hassall and Associates, Scott and Furphy and P.T. Indulexco, consultants. (1992) 'Annex 16: Women in Tourism', 'Annex 17: Small Scale Industry and Handicrafts', 'Annex 18: Education', 'Annex 19: Landuse.' Comprehensive Tourism Development Plan for Bali: Draft Final Report. United Nations Development Program, Government of the Republic of Indonesia.

Hermawati, P. and S. Kindon. (1993). *Gender Roles, Relations and Needs in the Balinese Development Process.* Student Publication Series Research Paper no. 14. Waterloo, Ontario: University Consortium on the Environment.

Hugo, G. J., T. H. Hull, V. J. Hull, G. W. Jones. (1990). *The Demographic Dimension in Indonesian Development.* Singapore: Oxford University Press.

Hyma, B. and S. Kindon. (1992). *A Review of the Bali Sustainable Development Project Village Surveys from a Gender Perspective.* University Consortium on the Environment Publication Series Research Paper no. 29. Waterloo, Ontario: University Consortium on the Environment.

Kindon, S., (ed.) (1993a). *Bali Sustainable Development Project: Gender and Development Training Workshop, June 22–23 1992.* University Consortium on the Environment Publication Series Research Paper no. 48. Waterloo, Ontario: University Consortium on the Environment.

—— (1993b). *From Tea Makers to Decision Makers: Applying Participatory Rural Appraisal to Gender and Development in Rural Bali, Indonesia.* University Consortium on the Environment Student Publication Series Research Paper no. 16. Waterloo, Ontario: University Consortium on the Environment.

Kinniard, V. and D. Hall (eds) (1994). 'Tourism: A Gender Analysis', Chichester, England: John Wiley & Sons Ltd.

Kinniard, V., Kothari, U. and Hall, D. (1994). 'Tourism: Gender Perspectives.' in *Tourism: A Gender Analysis*, eds V. Kinnaird and D. Hall. Chichester, England: John Wiley & Sons Ltd.

Koencaraninggrat. (1970). *Pengatar Anthropologi.* Jakarta: Penerbit Universitas.

Lansing, J. (1974). *Evil in the Morning of the World. Phenomenological Approaches to a Balinese Community.* Ann Arbor: The University of Michigan Center for South and Southeast Asian Studies.

Lee, W. (1991). 'Prostitution and Tourism in South-East Asia.' in *Working Women: International Perspectives on Labour and Gender Ideology*, eds N. Redclift and M. T. Sinclair. New York: Routledge.

Lim, N. Z. (1992). 'Women and Cultural Tourism: The Philippines Experience.' in *Universal Tourism Enriching or Degrading Culture*, eds J. Ave, J. Hillig and K. Hardjasoemantri. Yogyakarta, Indonesia: Gadjah Mada University Press.

Long, V. (1995). 'Community Characteristics and Tourism Development Impacts.' Doctoral dissertation. Unpublished dissertation draft: Department of Geography, University of Waterloo.

Long, V. and G. Wall. (1995). 'Small Scale Tourism Development in Bali.' in *Island Tourism: Management, Principles and Practice*, eds M. Conlin and T. Baum. Sussex, England: John Wiley & Sons Ltd.

Mabbett, H. (1987). *In Praise of Kuta*. Wellington, New Zealand: January Books.

McKean, P. F. (1989). 'Towards a Theoretical Analysis of Tourism: Economic Dualism and Cultural Involution in Bali.' in *Hosts and Guests: The Anthropology of Tourism*, (2nd ed.), ed. Valene L. Smith. Philadelphia: University of Pennsylvania Press.

McTaggart, W. (1980). 'Tourism and tradition in Bali.' *World Development* 8: 457–66.

Mantra, I. B. (1991). 'Tourism Industrial Impact on Socio-Cultural Life in Ubud, Bali.' Unpublished paper presented at the Bali Sustainable Development Project, third workshop, Bali, June 24–27.

Manuaba, I. B. A., T. I. Oka and I. K. Suwena. (1989). *Meningkatkan Mutu Kepariwisataan Di Uhud Dan Peliatan Melalui Perbiakan Kemampuan Pelayanan Dan Fasilitas Indsutri Serta Dukungan Penduduk*. Denpasar, Bali: Universitas Udayana.

Miller, D. and J. Branson. (1984). 'Pollution in Paradise: Hinduism and the Subordination of Women in Bali.' *Asian Studies Association of Australia Fifth National Conference*, University of Adelaide, May 13.

Moser, C. (1989). 'Gender Planning in the Third World: Meeting Practical and Strategic Gender Needs.' *World Development* 17: 1799–1825.

Noerhajati, S., I. Sutrilah, D. Sintaasih, M. Dewi, R. Wahyurini and G. Ekayana. (1993). in *Bali Sustainable Development Project: Gender and Development Training Workshop, June 22–23 1992*. University Consortium on the Environment Publication Series Research Paper no. 34. Waterloo, Ontario: University Consortium on the Environment.

Noronha, R. (1976). 'Paradise Reviewed: Tourism in Bali.' in *Tourism, Passport to Development?*, ed. E. De Kadt. New York: Oxford University Press.

Norris, J. (1994). 'Gender and Tourism in Rural Bali: A Case Study of Kedewatan Village.' Unpublished MA thesis: Department of Anthropology and Sociology, University of Guelph.

Ong, A. (1988). 'Colonialism and Modernity: Feminist Representation of Women in Non-western Societies.' *Inscriptions* 3/4: 79–93.

Picard, M. (1990). ' "Cultural Tourism" in Bali: Cultural Performances as Tourist Attraction.' *Indonesia* 49: 37–74.

—— (1993). 'Cultural Tourism in Bali: National Integration and Regional Differentiation.' in *Tourism in Southeast Asia*, eds M. Hitchcock, V. T. King and M. Parnwell. London: Routledge.

Richter, L. K. (1994). 'Exploring the Political Role of Gender in Tourism

Research.' in *Global Tourism: the Next Decade*, ed. W. F. Theobald. Oxford: Butterworth-Heinemann Ltd.

Rodenburg, E. E. (1980). 'The Effects of Scale in Tourism Development Tourism in Bali.' *Annals of Tourism Research* 7: 177–96.

Ruddick, A. (1986). 'Charmed Lives: Illness, Healing, Power and Gender in a Balinese Village.' Unpublished Ph.D. dissertation: Department of Anthropology, Brown University, Rhode Island, USA.

Sadli, S. (1992). 'Professionalization of Women in Cultural Tourism.' in *Universal Tourism Enriching or Degrading Culture*, eds J. Ave, J. Hillig and K. Hardjasoemantri. Yogyakarta, Indonesia: Gadjah Mada University Press.

Santosa, S. (1980). *Bali, What and Where*. Bali: Guna Agung.

—— (1985). *Gianyar, Valley of the Ancient Relics, Arts and Culture*. Gianyar, Bali, Indonesia: Regency Government of Gianyar, Bali, Indonesia.

SCETO. (1971). *Bali Tourism Study*. United Nations Development Program, International Bank for Reconstruction and Development.

Smith, D. (1987). *The Everyday World as Problematic*. Boston: Northeast University Press.

Smith, V. L. (1994). 'Privatization in the Third World: Small-scale Tourism Enterprises.' in *Global Tourism: the Next Decade*, ed. W. F. Theobald. Oxford: Butterworth-Heinemann Ltd.

Soebadio, H. (1992). 'Women and Cultural Tourism in Indonesia.' in *Universal Tourism Enriching or Degrading Culture*, eds J. Ave, J. Hillig and K. Hardjasoemantri. Yogyakarta, Indonesia: Gadjah Mada University Press.

Stringer, P. (1981). 'Hosts and Guests: The Bed and Breakfast Phenomenon.' *Annals of Tourism Research* 8: 357–76.

Suradiya, I. M. (1994). 'Batubulan and Celuk: Surprising Art and Craft Villages.' in *Bali*, ed. E. Oey. Singapore: Periplus Editions.

Suryakusuma, J. (1991). 'State Ibuism: The Social Construction of Womanhood in the Indonesian New Order.' *New Asian Visions* 6: 46–71.

Sutton, M. (1991). 'Knowledge, Governance and Tourism: Colonial Construction of Balinese Culture.' Paper presented at the Eighth Annual Berkeley Conference on South-East Asian Studies. Berkeley, California, February.

Swain, M. (ed.) (1995). 'Gender and Tourism,' special issue. *Annals of Tourism Research* 22: 2.

Thanh-Dam, T. (1983). 'The Dynamics of Sex-tourism: The Cases of Southeast Asia.' *Development and Change* 14: 533–53.

Thorbecke, E., T. van der Pluijm. (1993). *Rural Indonesia: Socio-economic Development in a Changing Environment*. New York: New York University Press.

Udayana State University Research Team. (1975). *The Impact of Tourism on Village Community Development*. Denpasar, Indonesia: State University of Udayana.

Universitas Gadjah Mada, Pusat Studi Wanita. (1993). *Peningkatan Peran Wanita Di Bidang Pariwisata*. Yogyakarta, Java, Indonesia: Universitas Gadjah Mada.

Universitas Udayana and Francillon, G. (1975). 'Tourism in Bali – its

Economic and Socio-cultural Impact: Three Points of View.' *International Social Sciences Journal* 27 (4): 721–5.

Wahnschafft, R. (1982). 'Formal and Informal Tourism Sectors: A Case Study in Pattaya, Thailand.' *Annals of Tourism Research* 9: 429–51.

Wall, G. (1990). 'Planning the Rate of Social Change: Bali, Indonesia.' Paper presented at the Caribbean Tourism Organization Conference on 'Tourism and Socio-cultural change in the Caribbean', Trinidad and Tobago, June.

Wall, G. (1993). 'Towards a Tourism Typology.' in *Tourism and Sustainable Development: Monitoring, Planning, Managing*, eds J. G. Nelson, R. Butler and G. Wall. Waterloo, Ontario: Department of Geography, University of Waterloo.

Wall, G. and V. Long. (1993). 'Beyond the Resorts: Balinese Excursion Routes and Land Use Change.' Paper presented at the 89th Annual Conference of the Asociation of American Geographers, Atlanta, Georgia, June.

Warren, C. A. (1990). 'Adat and Dinas: Village and State in Contemporary Bali.' Unpublished Ph.D. dissertation: Department of Anthrolpology, University of Western Australia.

Wiasti, M. (1989). *Peran Ganda Wanita Pedesaan – Studi Kasus Ibu Rumah Tangga Yang Berkerja di Sektor Formal dan Informal di Desa Pejaten*. Denpasar, Indonesia: Universitas Udayana.

Wiratmadja, A. (1991). *Wanita Hindu dalam Suatu Proyeksi*. Bandung, Indonesia: Ganesa Exact Bandung.

Chapter 6

Gender and tourism employment in Mexico and the Philippines

Sylvia Chant

INTRODUCTION

This chapter addresses gender differences in tourism and tourism-related employment in Mexico and the Philippines, with particular reference to women's work in international travel destinations. Core issues include the nature, conditions and earning capacities of key 'feminized' occupations, the reasons for gender segregation in tourism economies, and the implications of women's income-generating activity for household structure and survival among the poor. The chapter is also interested in exploring the often contradictory outcomes for women of work in international tourism resorts and the effects upon their status within the home and in wider society.

Mexico and the Philippines might seem unlikely countries to review in the same chapter given their substantially different economies and tourism industries, however what is striking in both contexts is the allocation of women to narrowly bounded (and often disadvantaged) niches in tourism labour markets. Possible reasons include the subordinate positions assigned to women by social and cultural constructions of gender in the two countries and the ways in which these, in turn, are embedded in, and often intensified by, contemporary development processes. With this in mind, the chapter commences with a brief overview of tourism in Mexico and the Philippines and provides a resumé of gender roles and relations among low-income groups, paying particular attention to the influences of wider economic and social change in recent years. Following this, detailed survey material from selected case study localities (Puerto Vallarta in Mexico, and Cebu and Boracay in the Philippines – see Figures 6.1 and 6.2)[1] illuminates various aspects of female employment and the outcomes for women and

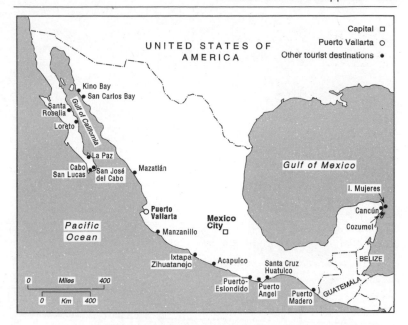

Figure 6.1   Mexico: location of Puerto Vallarta and other major tourist destinations

their households at the local level. The conclusion addresses the wider ramifications of women's participation in international tourism and points to areas in which the gains from this employment are most likely to be consolidated.

TOURISM IN MEXICO AND THE PHILIPPINES: AN OVERVIEW

While the economies of Mexico and the Philippines differ in a wide variety of ways, both rely heavily on tourism as a major source of export earnings[2] and are prominent destinations for international visitors, even if the Philippines has a much smaller share than Mexico of the international tourist market at the world and regional levels. For example, in 1990 the number of international tourist arrivals to the Philippines amounted to 893,000, representing only 4.1 per cent of the total visitors to Southeast Asia (WTO, 1992b: 137).[3] In the same year, Mexico was visited by 6,393,000 visitors from abroad, which was 39.1 per cent of all foreigners going to

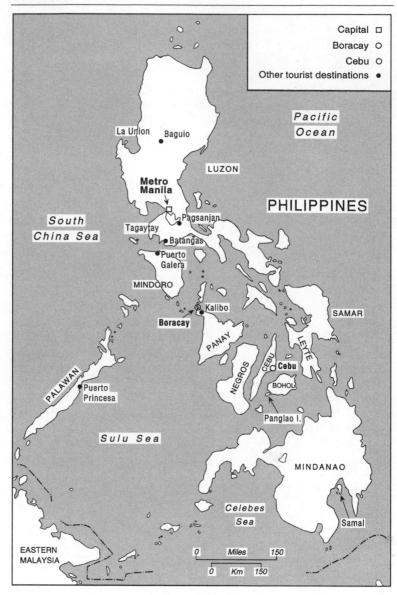

Figure 6.2   Philippines: location of Boracay, Cebu and other major tourist destinations

Latin America) (ibid.: 97). Reflecting these differences in numbers of tourist arrivals, receipts from international tourism are currently much smaller in the Philippines than Mexico: $1306 million US compared with $5342 million US in 1990 (ibid.: 108–112). Indeed, tourism in Mexico accounts for about 6 per cent of GDP and produces nearly 20 per cent of Mexico's non-oil foreign exchange (Barry, 1992: 151). Both countries are included in the World Tourism Organisation's list of top 60 world tourism destinations: on the basis of numbers of tourist arrivals in 1990, Mexico came seventeenth in the league table (Malaysia being the only 'non-advanced' economy ranking higher), with arrivals having grown at an average annual rate of 8.7 per cent since 1985 (well above the mean figure for all 60 countries of 6.7 per cent during this period). The Philippines, on the other hand, ranked fifty-second in 1990 and had a slower annual growth rate (3.4 per cent) between 1985 and 1990 (WTO, 1992b: 119). When considering rankings based on tourism receipts, however, both countries come out more favourably. Using this measure, Mexico's comes tenth in the league table with a total of 2.1 per cent of receipts worldwide, making it the highest-ranking non-industrialized country. The Philippines with 0.5 per cent of global tourism receipts also has a higher position – thirty-seventh. At the same time, with annual growth rates in tourism receipts of 12.9 per cent and 5.6 per cent between 1985 and 1990, neither of the countries came near the world average of 17 per cent per annum during this time (ibid.: 120).

One major difference between the tourism industries of the two countries relates to levels of provision of hotel accommodation. In 1990, Mexico's accommodation capacity was 333,547 rooms in hotels and similar establishments, whereas the equivalent in the Philippines was only 15,578 (WTO, 1992b: 147–8). This, in turn, reflects the high number of resort areas in Mexico compared with a relatively restricted range of Filipino destinations (see below). None the less, while Mexico undoubtedly is a world 'giant' in international tourism, the majority of its visitors are drawn from a rather narrow range of places. In 1987 for example, North Americans (from the United States and Canada) constituted 93 per cent of all tourists to Mexico from abroad (with a further 2.5 per cent from Europe and 4 per cent from the rest of Latin America) (EIU, 1991: 25). In the Philippines, on the other hand, the geographical origins of foreign tourists are much more diverse: in 1990 for example, only 23.1 per cent came from the USA and Canada, with nearly as many coming from Japan (19.7 per cent), and substantial numbers from Hong Kong (6.9 per cent), Taiwan (5.5 per cent) and Australasia (4.9 per cent) (WTO, 1992a: 201–2). By 1992, Japanese tourists had become the largest group, representing 20.1 per cent of arrivals between January and November that year; the USA and Canada's share had fallen to 18.9 per cent, but as many as 10.7 per cent came from Taiwan. Indeed, between November 1991 and November 1992, Taiwanese tourists to the Philippines increased from 4817 (5.4 per cent of all foreign visitors) to 12,204 (13.2 per cent of the total), representing a rise of 153 per cent (DOT, 1992). By 2010 it is expected that nearly two-thirds of international tourists will be from the Far East (Republic of the Philippines et al., 1991: 7, table 1)

In terms of recent trends in international tourism to the two countries, we can also detect elements of divergence. While Mexico has experienced a consistent increase in international visitors since the mid-1980s, the Philippine situation appears to be one of greater flux (see Table 6.1).

The downturn in Philippine tourism in 1990, however, does not seem to have endured. Amongst other things, the consistent efforts of the Department of Tourism to promote the industry and to bolster existing resorts means that there is likely to be at least a modest recovery in the present decade (see for example, NEDA, 1990).[4] Indeed, the Department of Tourism expects visitor arrivals to grow at a rate of 12.5 per cent over the next few years to reach a total of 1.7 million by 1996 (DOT, 1991b).

Growth in tourism in each country relies on rather different kinds of resources. While both Mexico and the Philippines offer conventional 'sun-and-sea' attractions, a major distinguishing factor for Mexico is its rich historical heritage, especially its pre-Columbian relics and abundant Spanish colonial architecture. While the Philippines by no means lacks sites of historical interest, a large element of international tourism is indubitably premised on the

Table 6.1 Trends in international tourist arrivals to Mexico and the Philippines, 1986–1990

| Country | Arrivals (thousands) | | | | |
	1986	1987	1988	1989	1990
Mexico	4625	5407	5692	6186	6393
The Philippines	764	781	1023	1076	893

Source: World Tourism Organization (1992b: 97–9).

country's contemporary 'hospitality' industry whereby lone men or groups of men seek young girls for paid sexual companionship.[5] The latter fact is evidenced by the disproportionate number of men taking 'holidays' in the country. For example, 79.3 per cent of all foreign visitors to the Central Visayan region of the Philippines, which comprises the provinces of Cebu, Bohol, Negros Oriental and Siquijor, in 1990 were male (UP AIT, 1990: 8) and, of all foreign visitors, as many as 41 per cent travelled alone, a further 37 per cent with friends, and only 15.3 per cent with spouses (ibid.: 18). At the national level, a joint report of the Philippine government, the United Nations Development Programme and the World Tourism Organization claims that the fact that over four-fifths of foreign visitors are male reflects the 'sex tourism stigma of the 1970s and 1980s' (Republic of the Philippines *et al.*, 1991: 143).

Although advertising and the promotion of hospitality services in established sex trade centres such as Manila, Cebu and Pagsanjan (see Figure 6.2, p. 122) has ostensibly been played down since the demise of Marcos in the mid-1980s, and current programmes are attempting to promote the Philippines as a 'wholesome travel destination' (NEDA, 1991: 242), the historical legacy of sex tourism is undoubtedly exacerbated by the fact that information about the ease of obtaining women and children is still available through numerous channels.[6,7] For example, large numbers of advertisements for what are effectively Philippine 'sex tours' continue to be printed in foreign men's magazines, and as recently as 1992 a national Filipino newspaper reported that feminists had attacked a Japanese publishing house for a travel publication which informed men as to where to obtain the best sex in Southeast Asia at the cheapest prices.[8] Moreover, even regular tourism literature within the Philippines contains more than oblique allusions to 'entertainment' attractions, viz. the opening lines of an article in a magazine published by the Department of Tourism's Regional Office in Cebu in 1991:

Mention Cebu and warm vivid images instantly fill one's mind. Fine sandy beaches, fantastic diving sites, five-star resorts, beautiful Cebuanas,[9] friendly hospitable people . . . sunny days and sultry nights.

(see Javier, 1991: 1)

The article concludes with the statement:

Cebu is many things – spectacular beaches . . . exciting nightlife with dozens of modern discos, hotels, restaurants and other entertainment facilities rivalling those found only in Manila and other key cities of the world.

(ibid.: 4)[10]

The reference to Manila is by no means incidental since, along with Bangkok, the Philippine capital has a long-standing reputation as an 'International Sex City' (Matsui, 1991: 70), and, as Aida Santos (1991: 48) points out, it is widely known that tourism in the Philippines 'has had for its main attraction and commodity the Filipino woman'.

Having identified some of the differences in international tourism in Mexico and the Philippines, it is important to bear in mind that the governments of both countries have played a major role in promoting the industry through the creation of local and national agencies, through the provision of finance and infrastructure and through overseas advertising. In addition, the Philippine Department of Tourism in 1990 tried to counteract negative publicity arising from the attempted coup and generalized political unrest (see note 4, p. 166) by providing travel incentives for overseas Filipinos as well as instigating an 'International Travel Programme' to host selected foreign groups connected with the travel trade and the media. In 1990 alone, 78 such groups were hosted (NEDA, 1991: 242). Within this general context of institutional support, other recent government initiatives have included the development or expansion of new beach centres, particularly Boracay in the Western Visayas,[11] Northern Palawan in Luzon, Panglao Island in the Central Visayas and Samal in the southern island group of Mindanao (see Figure 6.2, p. 122). The creation or expansion of new destinations is in part an attempt to counteract the rather *ad hoc* development of older resorts such as Puerto Galera, and to increase the Philippines' relatively underutilized beach resources. In part, it is perhaps also to generate interest in places which do not, as yet, possess the negative associations of established sex trade centres.

In Mexico, which has a much greater number of sun-and-sea destinations than the Philippines, the government has also created new beach resorts such as Cancún, Ixtapa-Zihuatanejo, San José del Cabo/Loreta and Santa Cruz Huatulco (Long, 1993; Torres, 1992, 1994), as well as playing a role in enhancing the attractions of existing ones such as Puerto Vallarta and Mazatlán (see Figure

6.1, p. 121; also Chant, 1992: 94). The government is also increasingly encouraging foreign investment in the development of the tourism infrastructure in Baja California on the US–Mexico border (Herzog, 1990).

GENDER IN MEXICO AND THE PHILIPPINES: AN OVERVIEW

Constructions of gender in Mexico and the Philippines are inevitably important in determining the manner in which women are incorporated into tourism labour markets. With this in mind, the following section reviews elements of gender roles and relations in the two countries which are likely to have a bearing on male–female employment differences and the outcomes of women's work for themselves and their households.

Gender divisions of labour

One fundamental similarity in gender roles between Mexico and the Philippines is the primary responsibility assigned to women for reproductive labour (child care and housework). Even where women are engaged in paid employment (and in both countries they are not an insignificant component of the registered labour force – see Table 6.2), they are still expected to undertake a major share of domestic tasks, either alone, or in conjunction with other

Table 6.2   Mexico and the Philippines: selected gender indicators

		Mexico	The Philippines
Women's share of total employment 1990 (%)[1]		29.5	36.3
Adult illiteracy 1990 (%)	– Total	13	10
	– Female[2]	15	11
Females as % of males in parliament 1990[3]		14	10
Total fertility rate*	– 1965	6.7	6.8
	– 1990[4]	3.3	3.7

Sources: [1]ILO (1993: Table 3A 'Employment'); [2]World Bank (1992: 218–9, Table 1 'Basic Indicators'); [3]UNDP (1992: 144–5, Table 9 'Female–Male Gaps'); [4]World Bank (1992: 270–1, Table 27 'Demography and Fertility')
Note: * Total fertility rate refers to the average number of children born to a woman if she lives until the end of her childbearing years

women in the household. This applies even in the Philippines where although men do participate in housework and play a role in looking after children (see Aguilar, 1991: 159; Bucoy, 1992: 36; PROCESS, 1993), this is not to the same degree or as regularly as women (for example, Hollnsteiner, 1991b: 27; Zosa-Feranil, 1984: 399). Indeed, men in both countries who do much to help their wives in the home earn themselves the pejorative terms of being *ander di saya* (under their wives' skirts) in the Philippines (Hollnsteiner, 1991b: 278) or *mandilones* (apron-wearers) in Mexico. Men are thus largely spared from domestic work and instead devote the majority of their time to executing the role of main breadwinner and to representing their households within the wider community (see Hollnsteiner, 1991a: 256).

The greater symbolic and actual attachment of women to domestic labour coupled with male primacy as breadwinners means that female employment is usually seen as a secondary activity by men and women alike, notwithstanding its often critical importance to household income. Women are generally situated in lower-paid and less prestigious jobs than their male counterparts, and, since they are viewed as working mainly to supplement their husbands' wages, they are also accorded low status and remuneration by employers. This is widely seen to be the case both in Mexico (see for example, Benería and Roldan, 1987; Chant, 1987, 1991; García *et al.*, 1983; LeVine, 1993: Chapter 3) and the Philippines (BWM, 1985; Eviota, 1988, 1991; Licuanan, 1991). Although among less-privileged groups in the Philippines, 'some approval and prestige' is accorded to women who play a part in generating household income (Hollnsteiner, 1991a: 266), Rhodora Bucoy (1992: 37) notes that there is 'still an ambivalent attitude towards working wives'. This, in turn, is 'indicative of the persistence of the traditional attitude that women's place is in the home' (ibid.).[12] Although recession in both countries over the last 10–15 years has given rise to some challenges to existing role models insofar as increased poverty has meant that women have often had to go beyond the bounds of their domestic duties to seek ways of generating income for their households (see, for example, Illo, 1989; Santos and Lee, 1989, on the Philippines; Chant, 1991: Chapter 6, 1993a, 1994b; García Colomé, 1990; González de la Rocha, 1988a; de Oliveira, 1990 on Mexico), there is scant evidence to suggest that men have taken on a correspondingly greater share of domestic labour to help compensate for their wives' new burdens (Chant,1994b; Gabayet and Lailson, 1990).

Household and family

The persistent division between male and female duties household level is important since in both societies there is ....ng pressure on women to get married and have children (see Hollnsteiner, 1991a; Licuanan, 1991, on the Philippines; Benería and Roldan, 1987; Chant, 1991; LeVine, 1993, on Mexico). With few roles for adult females beyond those narrowly prescribed by gender and familial ideologies, parents in the Philippines with unmarried daughters of 30 years or more will often encourage their daughters to 'lower their sights' *vis-à-vis* choice of partner so as not to become *matandong dalaga* (old maids) (Hollnsteiner, 1991: 254). While birth rates are lower than they were, fertility is still fairly high in both countries (see Table 6.2), and public provision of abortion ranges from being virtually unobtainable in Mexico to completely illegal in the Philippines (ISSA, 1991; Miralao, 1989; Reyes, 1992; Rubin-Kurtzman, 1987). One of the reasons for continued high fertility in both countries is that siring children is an important symbol of masculinity and, within prevailing structures of gender relations, women's scope for independent decision-making on childbirth is limited (Hollnsteiner, 1991b: 278; Moreno, 1982; Young, 1982; but see also PROCESS, 1993: 50).

In terms of household structure, nuclear units tend to be the most common residential arrangement for people, even if other forms such as extended households and women-headed structures exist (see Castillo, 1991; Chant and McIlwaine, 1995; Eviota, 1986; Illo, 1989; Medina, 1991; Shimuzu, 1991, on the Philippines; Benería and Roldan, 1987; Chant, 1985a, 1985b, 1991; García *et al.*, 1983; LeVine, 1993; Selby *et al.*, 1990, on Mexico). The preponderance of nuclear households is significant, at least in Mexico, in that when children are young, women have little scope to delegate domestic labour and childcare to other adults as they are wont to do in extended households and, for this reason, often end-up as full-time housepersons (see for example, de Barbieri, 1982; Chant, 1985a; also Brydon and Chant, 1993: 156–8).

The male–female divide between productive and reproductive labour is undoubtedly in part responsible for the greater share of men in household decision-making although, in the Philippine case, conflicting interpretations of domestic power are much in evidence. The Filipino household, for example, is often portrayed as more egalitarian than in other societies, with women regarded as having an especially important role in financial matters (see Church, 1986; Illo, 1989; Medina, 1991). The extent of women's role in the administration of household income is often such that Castillo (1991: 250) argues that Filipino women are more 'co-managers' than 'implementers of their husbands' wishes'. However, this view is disputed by many other writers (for example, Aguilar, 1988; Israel-Sobritchea, 1991; Sevilla, 1989), with Leonora Angeles (1990: 22) claiming that the incomes of most Filipino households are now so low that this does not make 'financial management a source of power, dominance or liberation for women'. Moreover, while women might well be 'keepers of the family purse', they are not in any position to refuse their husbands' requests for gambling or drinking money (PROCESS, 1993: 51).

Besides the debate over the relative importance of women's control over money in Filipino households, the general structure of the 'family-household' would still appear to be based on what Elizabeth Eviota (1992: 113) describes as a 'hierarchy of relations where the man is the head and the woman is the subordinate'. Eviota also asserts that the Filipino household is 'hardly a harmonious unit with a single common interest governed by complementary roles and needs' and maintains that within the family-household 'men unambiguously exercise direct power over women' (ibid.). In the face of the structural dominance of men in household decision-making, Filipino women are observed to resort to a number of what have been termed 'indirect means' to get their way, which may involve crying, sulking, arguing, going back to their parents' homes, neglecting their husbands' needs and so on (Hollnsteiner 1991a: 260). Because these strategies are occasionally successful, a woman is 'lulled into thinking that she really holds power in a manipulative sense, even when she does not' (ibid.). However, other commentators, notably Elizabeth King and Lita Domingo (1986: 12) liken the situation of Filipino women to an 'underworld matriarchy' whereby, although ostensibly there might appear to be a 'man's world', the women 'rule without anybody but themselves knowing it'. But again, as Eviota (1991: 162) points out, while many Filipino women may have 'behind-the-scenes' power, 'indirect influence does not compare with and cannot substitute for direct participation'.

In Mexico, too, men tend to dominate household decision-making, especially in situations where women are housewives in nuclear households with no personal resource base from their own employment on which to draw. In a 1986 study by the present author of low-income communities in three Mexican cities, it was found that nearly half the women interviewed in nuclear units had no scope to make expenditure decisions on anything but the barest essentials of household subsistence (Chant, 1991: 206; see also note 15, p. 167). Moreover, most women are still not able to go out to work without consulting husbands (Chant, 1993a, 1994b), even if recession has gone some way to increasing households' needs for extra income and *ipso facto* has contributed to some widening of women's margins for negotiation (ibid.; also, Arias, 1990).

Gender inequalities

Regardless of the ways in which decision-making is negotiated at the domestic level, one obvious indicator of male privilege in both Mexico and the Philippines is the tolerance of male sexual behaviour, both before marriage and outside marital relationships, compared with the expectations for women to be chaste spinsters and faithful wives. This syndrome is often referred to as 'sexual double standards' or the 'double standard of morality' (see Hollnsteiner, 1991a: 253; Medina, 1991: 99; also Yu and Liu, 1980: 64) and, while by no means confined to these two countries, appears to be particularly characteristic of situations where Spanish Catholicism has overlain existing cultures and promoted a female role model based on the Virgin Mary.[13] Part and parcel of this complex is the singular devotion of wife to husband and tolerance of male 'misdemeanours', which may involve acceptance of long-standing sexual attachments to other women. In Mexico for example, it is common for men to have a mistress with whom they share a symbolic *casa chica* (small house), at the same time as possessing a *casa grande* (big house) in which reside their wives and children. In the Philippines, too, many married men have a *kerida* or *kabit* (mistress/companion) (Medina, 1991: 107–8). Among lower-income groups in particular, the weakening of emotional bonds through successive philandering may culminate in male abandonment of wives (see Eviota, 1992: 153; Francisco, 1990; Hollnsteiner, 1991a, 1991b, on the Philippines; Arizmendi, 1980; Bridges, 1980; Chant, 1985b, on Mexico).

Other aspects of gender inequality in both countries include domestic violence towards women (Hollnsteiner, 1991a; Israel-Sobritchea, 1991; Nagot, 1991 on the Philippines; de Barbieri and

iveira, 1989; Chant, 1985b; González de la Rocha *et al.*, 1990
lexico). Indeed one study of a poor neighbourhood in Manila
aled that only the *absence* of wife-beating was interpreted by
women as signifying that their husbands loved them (Hollnsteiner,
1991a: 263), and research on urban areas in Cebu province demonstrated that out of every ten women, five or six had at one time or
another been victims of domestic violence (de la Cerna, 1992: 5).
Various authors have also noted that there is frequently greater love
between parents and children than between husbands and wives (see
Sala-Boza, 1982; Yu and Liu, 1980, on the Philippines; Lomnitz,
1977 on Mexico), with men often turning to their male friends for
adult companionship. In the Philippines, for example, the male
barkada (gang or drinking group) fulfils this function (Hollnsteiner, 1991b).

In terms of gender socialization there is evidence that daughters
and sons are increasingly given the same opportunities for education,
at least at elementary level (and even at high school level in the
Philippines). Male–female gaps in illiteracy have narrowed so substantially in recent years that they are currently negligible (see Table
6.2). However, girls in both countries are still expected to do more
around the home with the result that this can affect their energy for
(and commitment to) schoolwork. Moreover, as Patricia Licuanan
(1991: 16) points out with reference to the Philippines, women's
relatively high educational attainment still fails to be matched by
commensurate status in the labour market (see also Villariba, 1993:
8). There is also evidence to suggest that parents cultivate what is felt
to be girls' 'innate' sense of parental duty and, in encouraging them
to put family needs before their own, may constrain the personal
mobility of young women. For example, in a case study of out-
migration from a Visayan village, Donn Hart (1971) notes that
unmarried daughters were more willing and could be relied upon
to a greater extent to share their earnings with their families. Another
study by Cristina Blanc-Szanton (1990: 351) among the Ilonggo
population of Iloilo Province, Panay Island revealed that couples
often prefer their first-born to be female since daughters are regarded
as more helpful and reliable. Notwithstanding the general code of
sexual conduct for women in the Philippines, the importance of filial
duty among young women means that even hostessing is accepted
provided the earnings are used to help natal families (Whitam *et al.*,
1985: 149; also NCRFW, 1989: 140; Villariba, 1993: 20). Indeed,
comparatively high-paid female sex workers may well continue in

their occupations after marriage, with 'economic considerations overcoming the loss of status' (Blanc-Szanton, 1990: 353). This also applies to situations where a single woman becomes a mistress reliant on economic support from a married man: as Blanc-Szanton (1990: 352) observes, 'after an initial somewhat negative reaction by friends and relatives, she can be accepted back into the community, if the family welcomes her'.

As regards the effects of economic development on gender roles and relations in Mexico and the Philippines, it would appear that strategies to accelerate economic growth and to counteract the huge debt burdens borne by both countries have not only exploited existing gender inequalities but in several respects intensified them. As part and parcel of liberalization and adjustment programmes in recent years, for example, both Mexico and the Philippines have experienced an upsurge in foreign investment, with the expansion of multinational export-processing plants and a parallel increase in industrial sub-contracting drawing heavily on female labour. Women engaged in labour-intensive work in multinational factories or as piece-workers in their own homes work long days for low wages, often in appalling conditions, and have little scope (in the case of factory workers) to continue their employment after marriage and/or the birth of a child (see for example, Aldana, 1989; ILMS, 1984; Pineda-Ofreneo, 1987; Rosario, 1985, on the Philippines; Benería and Roldan, 1987; Iglesias, 1985, on Mexico). The vast bulk of female factory workers are accordingly young and have little prospect of upward occupational mobility. This is also true of sex tourism in the Philippines where female workers are again young (usually under 28 years of age) and their involvement in this employment offers little chance for economic or social ascendancy in later years. As Aguilar (1988: 15) notes:

It is apparent that the international division of labour has effectively multiplied the points of antagonism in the class and gender struggles, in this case assigning to Filipino women the role of highly expendable gendered and race-typed worker in the export and sex industries as well as in agri-business.

Female employment patterns

Aside from work in entertainment and export-manufacturing, Filipino women are generally found in commerce and services, often of an informal nature. In the urban areas of the Philippines, for example, women are commonly employed as maids, or are self-employed or unpaid family workers in petty retail and trading, the latter including hawking, peddling, street-vending or tending/managing small *sari-sari* stores (variety stores/corner shops) (see Bucoy, 1992; Eviota, 1986; Francisco, 1990; Francisco and Carlos, 1988; Mangahas and Pasalo, 1994). Similar patterns occur in Mexico where women's informal income-generating activities often revolve around the making and selling of foodstuffs such as *tortillas* (flat maize- or wheat-flour pancakes) or *elotes* (garnished corn cobs), or other 'domestic' skills such as sewing, washing and ironing, and child-minding (see Arizpe, 1982; Chant, 1987, 1991, 1994a; LeVine, 1993: 112–13).

Reflecting the general nature of women's roles and their relations with men in Mexico and the Philippines, and the frequent 'domestic' and/or low-prestige nature of female employment, women in tourism centres are often concentrated in informal commerce and in menial service work. In the Philippines they are also found in sexual services. The latter, in turn, relates to constructions of gender in other societies where the combination of gender-differentiated sexual morés together with privileged access by men to money, power and personal freedom means that international (and national) male demand for commoditized sex is both feasible and accepted (see for example, Azarcon de la Cruz, 1985). On top of this, the cost-differential between the advanced economies and a developing country such as the Philippines provides what Hall (1992: 66) terms a 'drawcard to sex tourists'.[14]

Leaving sex work aside, however, while there are some similarities in the gendering of tourism employment in the two countries, there are also certain differences. On one hand, the limited case study literature available suggests that commerce is a major employer of women in both contexts, and that there are often interesting gender differences in scale of enterprise and the types of goods and services traded by male and female workers. For example, a study by Olofson and Cristosomo (1989) of two Philippine beach resorts in Cebu province: Panagsama Beach and Argao, found that women were predominantly engaged in the selling of shellcraft and manicures, whereas men were in the comparatively well-paid occupations of *bangkero* (boatman) and pedicab driver. This separation of male–female products and services is mirrored in divisions found in the Mexican tourist resort of Puerto Vallarta where female vendors tend mainly to trade in light, relatively low-cost items such as hand-made tablecloths, clothing, and fruit and other comestibles, with men primarily involved in the sale of heavier or more expensive products such as silverware, baskets, woven rugs and carpets, and hand-painted pottery, as well as providing services such as boat rides and personalized city tours (see Chant, 1991: Chapter 3).

However, in service establishments, differences between the countries are apparent. While in Mexican tourist resorts women are commonly employed as hotel chambermaids and laundry workers (see Chant, 1991: Chapter 3; Kennedy *et al.*, 1978; Reynoso y Valle and de Regt, 1979), in the Philippines, it is usually men who prevail in these positions. For example, a report by Lee (1981) indicates that in Manila hotels, most room cleaners and laundry workers are male, with one of the functions of room boys being to procure hospitality girls for guests. Indeed, the informal 'sexual service' sector attached to hotels is heavily reliant on male intermediaries and would arguably function less effectively with female brokers. Another possible reason is that offered by Ron O'Grady (1983: 11) who notes that foreigners visiting the Philippines are so accustomed to viewing local women as sexual objects that they often behave improperly to those who service their rooms and for this reason management have to substitute male for female workers.

In light of the relative dearth of studies of gender and tourism employment in Mexico and the Philippines, the following case studies aim to illuminate some of the male–female divisions in tourism employment in key localities and to highlight the major consequences for low-income women and their households. The bulk of the information about women is based on a combination of questionnaires and in-depth interviews (in which the author was the sole or co-interviewer) with women in a wide variety of occupations in the case study areas (see note 1, p. 165), and where considerable time and effort was devoted to building-up a rapport with respondents. In Mexico in particular, where the author has been able to conduct longitudinal work, strong relationships have developed with a number of women with whom contact has been maintained in the intervals between field visits (see also note 15, p. 167). The insights gained in these cases have added valuable perspectives to those gleaned from routine survey work, especially in respect of the changes in women's personal and home lives which have accompanied shifts in employment within the tourist industry.

FEMALE EMPLOYMENT IN PUERTO VALLARTA: A CASE STUDY

Puerto Vallarta is one Mexican resort which does not owe its origins to government initiative, even if the state has participated in various phases of its development since its initial establishment as a tourist destination some 30 years ago. Originally a small fishing village contained within a predominantly agricultural hinterland, Puerto Vallarta now has a population of around 250,000 and first came to major international attention in the early 1960s when John Huston chose it as the setting for his film of Tenessee Williams' *The Night of the Iguana*. The film starred Richard Burton who was visited on location by Elizabeth Taylor; this gave the town something of a romantic mystique and enhanced its attraction amongst North American visitors. Shortly afterwards, the Mexican government began intervening to create the necessary infrastructure for tourism expansion, including the building of a major road link to the western Pacific highway, the construction of an international airport and the establishment of a major regional planning agency to monitor and oversee development and, in particular, to regulate land occupation (see Chant, 1991: Chapter 2, 1992).

From 1970 onwards, demographic growth proceeded at a dramatic pace, averaging about 12 per cent per annum during the 1970s and first part of the 1980s. Growth was so impressive that, by the late 1980s, the construction of a major Marina development was underway some four miles north of the traditional town centre, with numerous new hotels, restaurants and commercial establishments springing up along the connecting highway. Most international tourists have traditionally come from the USA and Canada, especially during the dry season from October through to March, with large numbers of national tourists filling-in during the rainy period, especially in July and August when Mexican schoolchildren have their long vacation (see Chant, 1991: Chapter 2). However, the deteriorating dollar:peso exchange rate and the recession in the United States from the late 1980s onwards has reduced international demand relative to Puerto Vallarta's expanded capacity with the result that, at the beginning of the 1990s, the town was experiencing something of a crisis. While high-season occupancy of hotel rooms was as much as 100 per cent in the mid-to-late 1980s, by 1992 it was only 60–70 per cent. Even low season occupancy dropped from around 75 per cent to only 45 per cent over the same period

(Chant, 1994b). These problems are exacerbated by the fact that foreign and national visitors alike have less money to spend during their stay.

Although the town's population continues to grow, and Puerto Vallarta received at the beginning of the 1990s almost as many visitors by air as in the mid-1980s (around 1.5 million national and foreign visitors per annum), local people face declining opportunities for employment, and the income to be made from independent and/or informal entrepreneurial activity is now drastically reduced (see Chant, 1994b for a fuller discussion). This seems to have impacted on men to a greater extent than women although, while women may have been able to retain their access to work, they are still found in the lower rungs of the local labour market hierarchy. Reasons for the gender-differentiated nature of job losses possibly include the fact that the construction industry, a major employer of men, has been hardest hit by the crisis of over-investment. In addition, many men are unwilling to accept low-paid jobs which have traditionally been designated as 'female'.

Looking more closely at gender differences in employment in Puerto Vallarta, a detailed survey by the author in 1986 of low-income households and key local employers[15] revealed that while the three main sectors of tertiary employment in the city – commerce, catering and hotels – all employed women as well as men, women generally made up a lower proportion of the workforce, were usually in less prestigious positions, earned less money and had fewer opportunities for upward occupational mobility (see Chant, 1991: Chapter 3).

At the top of the employment hierarchy, 8 out of 21 firms in which interviews were undertaken by the author had a female personnel manager, but the average proportion of female employees in general was only just over one-third (37.4 per cent) (see Chant, 1991: 67, Table 3.1a). In terms of the sub-sectors, commerce was the only one where women were a majority workforce (66.2 per cent of workers in the six commercial establishments in the survey) (ibid.). This is partly because formal educational qualifications are generally deemed less important in determining eligibility for saleswork than personal/moral attributes such as honesty and trustworthiness (Chant, 1991: 72). At the same time, in more specialist retail enterprises such as silver shops, ability to speak English (which generally hinges on having some secondary schooling) is becoming increasingly important and tends to favour men who are more likely to be given the opportunity for post-primary education by their parents and/or to have greater freedom than their sisters to spend time as migrant workers in the USA. Generally speaking, however, commerce was found to be the one sector where there were greater possibilities for women to substitute for men. This was much less the case in hotels and restaurants where gendered niches of activity were very apparent.

Within the total of nine catering establishments included in the 1986 survey, which ranged from small snack bars to large exclusive restaurants, women amounted to only 25 per cent of workers (Chant, 1991: 67, Table 3.1a). Moreover, moving up the hierarchy of establishments, opportunities for women generally diminish. For example, in the five smallest restaurants and eateries in the sample (which cater for locals and tourists), women were as many as 71.4 per cent of employees, whereas they were only 18.2 per cent of workers in the top four establishments surveyed (two medium-sized and two large restaurants catering mainly for foreign tourists). In these top four establishments there was considerable evidence of gender segregation. The small number of women workers were employed mainly as secretaries and cashiers, and in only one establishment were they part of the kitchen staff (and then employed as dishwashers and kitchen hands rather than as cooks or chefs). There were no women at all in these four restaurants who served at table. Reasons given by personnel managers included the fact that top class restaurants worldwide tend to use waiters as opposed to waitresses, and it was felt that women might 'lower the tone' of these establishments. Another justification was that it was problematic to have men and women working alongside each other due to the likelihood of sexual and emotional liaisons developing among staff. As one manager put it 'el hombre es el fuego y la mujer es la broza' ('man is fire and women are the brushwood'). By keeping women restricted to 'female-only' areas such as cashiering, the intention is thus to reduce the prospect of complications of this nature arising (see Chant, 1991: 82).

This latter concern also figured in rationalizations for the segregation of male and female employees in hotels. Overall, women are a higher proportion of hotel staff (38.5 per cent in the 1986 survey of six hotels), but distinctions between men's and women's sections are rather rigidly demarcated. While posts in reception, offices and other areas requiring a secondary school education and/or vocational training seem relatively flexible in their recruitment patterns, among non-administrative workers, women are largely confined to house-keeping activities such as chambermaiding, linen-keeping and laundry work, whereas men are found across a much wider range of departments including portering, gardening, transport, and restaurant, kitchen and bar work.

This horizontal segregation between the male and female workforce is important for a number of reasons. First, it reflects (and in several respects reinforces) the traditional association of women with reproductive chores such as washing and bed-making, and that of men with 'heavier' duties, 'outside work' or work with a more 'public' orientation. Indeed, certain hotel managers claimed that interacting with customers in bars and restaurants was not suitable for women given the connotations surrounding hostessing and its perceived association with prostitution (Chant, 1991: 78). A second and related implication of gender segregation in hotel work is that many jobs that males perform are, by virtue of their public nature, likely to reap greater earnings. Although the basic wages of male and female service workers are often comparable (ibid.: 77, Table 3.5), bell-boys and porters, drivers, waiters and barmen tend to be much more directly involved with clients than female chambermaids and laundryworkers, with the result that gratuities are often more substantial. Indeed, some male employees receive up to five times as much as their basic wage from tips alone (ibid.: 76–7).

A third consequence of gender segregation in hotel employment and, in particular, the small number of 'female' sectors is limited occupational mobility. Unlike men who often achieve upward mobility by strategic 'sideways' moves into other sectors, women are more restricted to waiting for posts to become vacant in their own departments. In turn, female departments tend not to have a wide range of ranks and specializations, which means that women have to wait longer for promotion. To give an example, the only higher-status position to which a chambermaid can aspire is that of *ama de llaves* (housekeeper) (or deputy housekeeper if a department is large enough to sustain two supervisors). Such a move might take 10–15 years to attain, if at all, with most large hotels having one housekeeper for every twenty chambermaids. In contrast, in restaurant work there are possibilities for male kitchen hands to move into the dining area which, in turn, has an elaborate range of posts ranging from commis waiter (a 'runner' operating between the kitchen and serving staff), to full waiter, section waiter, wine waiter, chief waiter and even to restaurant supervisor and/or manager. Most men entering at low levels can expect some kind of promotion within a three-to-four year period. A related consideration is that it is rare for women to end up supervising a predominantly male section due to the perceived difficulties of men taking orders from women (Chant, 1991: Chapter 3).

Having perhaps provided a rather bleak outline of women's involvement in tourism employment in Puerto Vallarta, it is also important to point out that the mere fact that women have *access to work* is itself significant, especially at the household level. Comparative research by the author in two other Mexican cities – the industrial towns of León and Querétaro – in 1986 (see note 15, p. 167), revealed that women's labour force participation was much higher in Puerto Vallarta (Chant, 1991: 136, Table 4.8). This is mainly because tourist resorts are characterized by a large service sector where demand for female labour is high and because of the existence of feminized niches within hotel and restaurant work where women's assumed 'domestic' skills' give them an advantage over men (see also Kennedy *et al.*, 1978 on the Mexican resort of Ixtapa-Zihauatanejo and Torres, 1994 on Cancún).

One notable outcome of women's greater perceived and actual access to employment in Puerto Vallarta (also documented for other centres in Mexico and Latin America where women have above-average entry to the labour force such as the US–Mexico border and Puerto Rico – see Fernández-Kelly, 1983; Safa, 1981), is the high number of female-headed households in the locality. According to the author's survey among low-income households, as many as 19.6 per cent of households in Puerto Vallarta are headed by women compared with only 13.5 per cent in Querétaro and 10.4 per cent in León.[16]

This high proportion of female-headed households in Puerto Vallarta is very much related to employment. On one hand, because tourism offers a range of female job opportunities, lone women, with or without children, who may lack access to the means of survival in other places, are attracted to resort towns. At another level, the scope to earn an independent (and often reasonable and/or guaranteed) income means that there is not the same pressure on women to unite with men or remain with existing partners as in places where they have a less favourable position in the labour market. Indeed, it is instructive to note that formal marriage rates among women with co-resident male partners in the survey settlements in Puerto Vallarta are substantially lower (at 79.7 per cent) than in both Querétaro (91.6 per cent) and León (97.1 per cent) (Chant, 1991: 172–3), and many women talked of 'trying their men out' before they committed themselves; some also spoke of having 'booted-out "bad men"' in the past. Other factors which might account for the comparatively low incidence of formal marriage and co-residential sexual unions in Puerto Vallarta is that the resort only became a major area of in-migration in the 1970s and many people have not yet re-established their full kinship networks in town. Arguably this has allowed women a little more freedom from usual pressures to marry and/or to conform with socially expected norms. Another factor is that women in Puerto Vallarta come face-to-face with other cultures and practices and many comment not only on the generally more relaxed attitudes towards men and marriage among foreigners, but seem also to have adopted less conservative behaviour themselves. For example, unlike their counterparts in the highland cities of León and Querétaro, most women dress casually (often in shorts and sleeveless T-shirts in the style of female tourists), are open about their relationships with men, and seem to be more forthcoming about their grievances concerning the opposite sex (both within the domestic context itself and to outsiders). Beyond this, lone mothers frequently encourage their daughters to postpone marriage and babies until a time when they have finished studying and/or established themselves economically. As expressed by one 34-year-old single parent, Guadalupe, who had raised three children more-or-less single-handedly, her main concern was that her 18-year-old daughter, Giovana, would be able to 'defenderse' (defend herself), and tourism resorts, in her opinion, tended to provide above average opportunities to do this (see below; also Chant, 1992: 98).

Aside from the existence of female-headed households, another corollary of women's access to employment is that women in male-headed households appear to have more egalitarian relationships with their spouses than in other parts of Mexico. This is especially the case for those in paid work and, again, arguably relates to the potential for these women to break away and form independent households of their own: in other words, men have to 'tow the line' or their wives might leave them (see also Chant, 1994b). The case of a 39-year-old cook, Dolores, who had come to Puerto Vallarta as a teenage bride and who, since then, had had a virtually unbroken run of work, is illustrative here. Dolores explained that her elderly husband (with whom there was an age gap of over 30 years), was no longer of any significant economic use, relied on her for everything, and had long let her have the upper hand in household afffairs, even to the extent of permitting her to have other sexual liaisons. As Dolores herself put it '*Yo soy el hombre y la mujer en esta casa – yo dirigo todo*' ('I am the man and the woman in this house – I'm in charge of everything') (see Chant,1991: 165). While not all women are able to exert such power within marital relationships, and personal characteristics undoubtedly come into the equation, it is interesting that this kind of pattern is much rarer in parts of the country where women's access to paid work and earnings is less (see for example, Chant, 1985b; González de la Rocha, 1988b)

A final, and broadly 'positive', consequence of women's access to work in Puerto Vallarta is that daughters of working women appear to be following in their mothers' footsteps insofar that they to tend to be participating in the workforce, and indeed often aspiring to and/or achieving higher positions in the labour market. A follow-up study conducted by the author among ten households in low-income settlements in Puerto Vallarta in 1992 indicated that some daughters here were entering higher education and/or had professional careers (see note 15, p. 167). This was in stark contrast to the findings of parallel follow-up studies in Querétaro and León where no daughter at all had entered tertiary education and only a handful had non-manual and/or skilled jobs. In turn, there appeared to be consistent links between work and marriage. Although by no means conclusive, the data gathered in Puerto Vallarta in 1992 suggested that girls were not getting married and/or having their first child until substantially later than in the industrial towns of León and Querétaro (see Chant, 1994b).

At the same time as there would appear to be certain advantages to women accruing from residence (and employment) in Mexican tourist resorts, it is also important to bear in mind that some men cannot seem to cope with their wives' or partners' economic independence and may 'retaliate' by either dropping out of work or scaling down their contributions to household income. In addition, some husbands in this position even use their wives' earnings to play cards or to go out drinking with male friends. Another important issue is that women who work outside the home are usually still left with the majority of domestic tasks, either to carry out alone or in conjunction with other household members (generally female kin or daughters).

Whether these patterns will persist will depend on a number of factors. In the wake of the economic crisis which has hit Puerto Vallarta since the beginning of the 1990s, it seems that a greater number of husbands and sons are unemployed while women have maintained their hold on waged work and indeed in some cases have moved upwards in the employment hierarchy in terms of position or earnings (Chant, 1994b). If unable to increase their returns from a single job, one way in which women have sustained their earning power is through diversifying their income-generating activities. For example, one 34-year-old mother of two, Fildelina, who in 1986 had been doing hair-cutting on a part-time basis in her own home had, by 1992, both converted her front room into a retail outlet and taken a job as a domestic servant. Another respondent, Elba, who was a domestic servant in 1986, has since supplemented her income by selling bags of ice from her kitchen fridge (see Chant, 1994b). Men on the other hand, even if unemployed, have tended to keep their sights set on formal employment, rather than diverting their efforts into informal and/or domestic-based income-generation. Nor is there much evidence for an upturn in the amount of unpaid work they might do around the home such as housework and child-minding. This asymmetry in male–female inputs into family life could conceivably result in further fragmentation of household units if the crisis persists (see Benería, 1991). There is also the danger that women's labour market gains in tourist resorts such as Puerto Vallarta will be cancelled out by serious erosion of their time and energy as the burdens of working in and outside the home remain unrelieved by any assistance on the part of men.

FEMALE EMPLOYMENT IN CEBU AND BORACAY: A CASE STUDY

In contrast to Puerto Vallarta, both the Philippine case study localities are undergoing expansion. While the two resorts are rather different, between them they combine most aspects of tourism in Puerto Vallarta. Boracay, on the one hand, is a quiet sun-and-sea destination which attracts a lot of 'backpackers' and where informal employment in commerce and services exists alongside a fairly small-scale formal sector. Cebu, on the other hand, caters more for business visitors and organized tours, and most workers are in large-scale registered establishments.

Cebu City

Cebu City is capital of Cebu province, is the second most important city in the Philippines after the capital, Manila, and has a population of around 650,000. While Cebu is primarily an industrial, shipping and commercial centre, it is also an important destination for international tourism, ranking second in the country after Manila (see NEDA Region VII, 1992; Republic of the Philippines, 1990).[17] In terms of the Philippine Tourism Master Plan, Cebu (and Boracay) form part of the so-called 'Visayas Cluster' whereby visitors are encouraged to take advantage of easy access and special-rate trips to tourist spots in other parts of the region such as Panglao Island, Bohol, Bacolod City in Negros Oriental, and Iloilo City on Panay Island (DOT, 1991b; Republic of the Philippines et al., 1991).

The origins of tourism in Cebu date back to the early 1980s. Various beach resorts have been built on the island of Cebu itself and the adjacent island of Mactan, which is connected by a road bridge as well as a regular ferry service and which forms part of the Cebu metropolis.[18,19] Much construction has been financed by foreign, especially Japanese, investment and the city of Cebu itself is host to numerous international visitors, many of whom have business interests in the locality. Estimates suggest that business-men (as opposed to women) make up around 40 per cent of all foreign visitors. This is viewed as healthy by the Cebu Chapter of the Hotel, Restaurant and Resort Association, since a large business visitor component tends to stabilize demand in an otherwise fairly sensitive market. Indeed it is revenue from this segment which local tourism agencies are trying to increase by encouraging businessmen to extend their stays and make use of facilities such as guided city tours, water sports and so on.[20]

In 1990, Cebu received 304,902 tourist arrivals per annum; just over one-third of these (120,000) were from abroad, representing 13.4 per cent of all foreign visitors to the Philippines (UP AIT, 1990: 2). By 1992 numbers of foreign visitors to Cebu had increased to 131,859. The vast bulk of visitors are from Japan (50,000 in 1991), but the USA, Taiwan and Hong Kong also figure prominently (13,000 US visitors arrived in Cebu in 1991, 10,000 from Taiwan and 8000 from Hong Kong) (Mackie, 1992: 80). The flow of Japanese tourists has been enhanced by the introduction of a twice-weekly direct flight between Tokyo's Narita Airport and Cebu's nearby Mactan Island International Airport, and many come to Cebu for as little time as a weekend given that it is actually cheaper to pay for a golfing package than it is to play at home (ibid.). There are also four direct flights a week between Mactan and Hong Kong, twice a week to and from Singapore, while flights to other key destinations such as Taipei (Taiwan) and Seoul (South Korea) are available through link services via Manila whereby all customs, immigration and luggage procedures are handled in Cebu.

Though some visitors are attracted to Cebu's sun-and-sea resorts, the character of tourism in Cebu is predominantly business-related and urban, and the city-based 'entertainment' industry is undoubtedly a major factor in accounting for recent growth in international arrivals (see de la Cerna, 1992: 53). Indeed, the entertainment sector is likely to expand considerably in the current decade due to the projected (and actual) influx of sex workers displaced from US base areas in the northern island group of Luzon. Until August 1991 when Mount Pinatubo erupted and destroyed the surrounding area, one of the two major installations, Clark Air Base, provided high demand for 'hospitality' services in the neighbouring city of Angeles; this was also the case with Olongapo, home to the US 7th Fleet until the end of 1992. Although there are plans on the part of Olongapo's mayor, Richard Gordon, to convert the former base into an international Hong Kong-style duty-free shopping, service and light manufacturing centre (see EIU, 1993: 16–17), many women have already started leaving the city. Indeed, a national newspaper noted that between 1990 and 1991 alone, when people first started departing the base areas, the number of registered commercial sex workers in Cebu rose by as much as 20 per cent.[21] In 1992, the City Health Office reported a total of 1557 commercial sex workers attending compulsory routine check-ups, although this by no means included all women working in the trade (de la Cerna, 1992: 53).[22] Despite Cebu's attempt, in the words of the Vice President of the local chapter of the Hotel, Restaurant and Resort Association, to promote Cebu as 'an island in the Pacific' as a means of shaking-off the sex tour image of Manila and Pagsanjan, demand by foreigners for sexual services has been on the increase since the early 1980s when a major protest about the exploitation of Filipino women took place in Manila and resulted in the transfer of Japanese sex tourists away from the limelight of the capital to Cebu (see Azarcon de la Cruz, 1985: 26; Matsui, 1991: 71–2).

Hotel employment

Not all workers in tourism establishments in Cebu are obviously engaged in the hospitality sector *per se*, although 'conventional' tourism establishments have substantially lower proportions of female employees. A survey by the author of four major hotels in Cebu with a total of 1261 workers between them, for example, showed that only 39 per cent of employees were women.[23] While this figure is comparable to similar surveys in the hotel industry in Puerto Vallarta, it is low compared with the proportion of women in other types of employment in Cebu, such as export-manufacturing, where women make up around three-quarters of workers (see Chant and McIlwaine, 1995: Chapter 4), and the entertainment industry where they are nearer 90 per cent (see below).

The proportion of women working in Cebu hotels would probably be higher were it not for the fact that what are exclusively or significantly 'female domains' in Mexico are 'mixed sex' departments in the Philippines. For example, housekeeping departments, which in Mexican hotels are 100 per cent female, are only 40 per cent female in Cebu. Housekeeping staff in Cebu's hotels consist of bed-makers, room boys (who perform the general cleaning of rooms), housemen (who clean public areas such as corridors, lobbies and so on), laundry workers and linen keepers. While women sometimes make beds, room-cleaning is generally a male preserve – the rationale ostensibly being that strength is needed to shift furniture. This also applies to housemen, and in some cases to bed-making itself. However, as suggested earlier, reasons less likely to be stated include the fact that pervasive notions of Filipina women as sexual objects can result in harrassment of maids in the intimate context of hotel bedrooms and, more insidiously, that male guests are more likely to approach male employees for sexual contacts; by placing men in room jobs therefore, hotels are conceivably able to offer information on sexual entertainment in an 'undercover' fashion. As far as food and beverage departments are concerned, some large hotels use women as 'food attendants' (mainly because they are 'pleasing to customers'), but women are rarely to be found in kitchen work, the rationale being that much of this is mechanized. The use of large industrial dishwashers, for example, is common, and men are thought to have more of an affinity with machinery.

The only sections in hotels in which women are found in significant numbers are administration and accounts (49 per cent female), and, at lower levels, in front desk duties as receptionists, cashiers and telephone operators (45 per cent). Again, women would probably represent a greater proportion of staff in the latter were it not for the fact that porters and bellboys are generally included in these numbers and that male desk clerks are employed to do the overnight or 'graveyard' shift (it being against the law to employ women for nightwork except in cases where activities are deemed specifically to require female workers – see Chant and McIlwaine, 1995). Employers mentioned the value of having women on the front desk because of their charm, patience and physical attractiveness, all deemed assets in an environment where the majority of guests are foreign and/or Filipino businessmen. A situation pertains, therefore, in which women in formal hotel employment tend to be favoured for jobs with a strong above-board 'liaison' component, predicated, in turn, on images of Filipino women as objects of male desire and gratification (see Chant and McIlwaine, 1995: Chapter 5).

The employment of men in jobs which display a much closer association with stereotypical female roles in the Philippines (such as cooking, cleaning and kitchen work), on the other hand, is interesting, and aside from those posts where men have a potential role in sexual brokerage may, in part, be due to the fact that Filipino men are not as unaccustomed to housework as they are in many other countries. At another level, it might have to do with the fact that all hotel employment has a privileged status in a situation of limited formal sector opportunities.[24] Where employers can afford to be highly selective, as is the case in Cebu, men might be recruited not only because of pervasive notions that men 'need' work more women, but also because they are likely to be better-educated. Certainly a high level of education is required even for non-administrative posts in hotels, with most employees being high school, if not college graduates.[25] This is mainly because only educated people speak sufficient English to be able to communicate with foreign guests. As for the privileged status of hotel work, while most employees earn no more than the daily wage of those in factories and shops (i.e. the legal minimum rate of only P105 or $4.20 US), supplements from service charges and tips mean that take-home pay is considerably higher. All non-administrative staff in Cebu's hotels receive a share of a 10 per cent service charge levied on rooms, food and drink. In firms with strong unions, non-administrative workers may receive the whole of the service charge; in others, the proportion is 85 per cent with 15 per cent going to management (part of which is used to cover breakages). Each individual's share of the service charge can often amount to P1500 ($60.50) a week, more than twice the average weekly wage of P630 ($25.20) as of 1993. While the service charge is distributed evenly among workers, tip systems vary from place to place. Generally speaking those in food and and beverages receive the most (perhaps between P50–500 [$2–20 US] a day), whereas those cleaning rooms receive very little, mainly because it is not the custom for Filipino guests to tip their cleaners. Moreover, those on the front desk performing clerical and telephone duties (as opposed to 'bellhops' or porters) usually earn no tips at all. On average then, just as in Mexico, female hotel employees are generally in departments with the lowest levels of gratuities. It is in the hospitality sector, however, that women can and do make reasonable earnings, and where they are certainly the bulk of the workforce.

Hospitality work

Cebu City has several establishments which offer so-called 'night-time pleasures'. Aside from brothels (*casas*), which tend to be patronized by local people or Filipino visitors to Cebu (and which tend to be Filipino-owned), formal hospitality establishments range from discothèques which feature semi-nude dancers, to those with thematic floor shows, to the increasingly popular karaoke bars where men sing along to Western songs accompanied by young, attractive 'guest relations ladies' (hostesses). Most common, however, are the so-called 'girlie bars' where people sit drinking around a stage watching a constant stream of bikini- or underwear-clad performers ('back-to-back models'), and can 'bar fine' those they wish to take out of the establishment. The latter involves paying a fee to the club owner or manager to release the employee concerned for a specified period (usually the rest of the night). While karaoke bars are normally run by Japanese businessmen (often in association with the Yakuza),[26] girlie bars tend to be the property of Australians, North Americans or West Europeans who almost invariably have Filipino wives[27] (see also Moselina, 1981: 24–5 on Olongapo; Wilke, 1983: 15 and WRRC/PSC, 1990: 5 on Manila). Although men are also employed in the establishments, it is usually as door-men, bar attendants and floor managers (*papasan*). In other words, men's bodies are not generally for sale, even if they are occasionally propositioned by customers.[28] Women, on the other hand, usually work as dancers, 'guest relations ladies' and receptionists, and only rarely have the opportunity to become bar attendants or *mamasan* (female floor managers) (see Chant and McIlwaine, 1995: Chapter 6).

Unlike hotel employment, education is not necessarily a prerequisite for entry, although women normally have to have gone through high school in order to be able to converse with foreign customers. At the same time, a minority without foreign language skills may start as dancers and gradually pick up English or Japanese as they go on. In one sense educational qualifications present something of a contradiction in that it slows up the entry into the business of young (pre-high school graduate) teenagers who tend to be extremely popular among clients: foreign and Filipino customers alike are more interested in ogling the women than conversing with them, and also regard younger girls as being 'fresher' (more energetic, less jaded by extensive sexual activity), and 'cleaner' (less likely to have STDs or to be HIV-positive) (see Chant and McIlwaine, 1995: Chapter 6). None the less, with rising numbers of Filipinos gaining access to further and higher education, and through fear of recruiting under-age workers, employers in the more prestigious establishments are now tending to sacrifice youth in favour of academic credentialism. For example, one advertisement for a vacancy in the karaoke section of an up-market Japanese restaurant in Cebu's main local paper *Sun Star Daily* on 6th April 1993, ran:

> Criteria for applicants: pretty, at least 5'2" tall, college level, pleasing personality and conversant in English and a little knowledge of Nippongo.

Notwithstanding a preference for teenage women among clients, the average age of nightclub hostesses (including dancers and chat-up girls) tends to be between 22 and 27. Good looks and a lithe body are critical and, in cases where women are extremely 'well-preserved', they can even go on working after childbirth and into their early 30s. In a worker interview sample it transpired that the vast majority of respondents despised what they did but were there through lack of alternative employment (or such well-remunerated employment – see below) and/or because they had children to raise alone. Indeed, ten out of fourteen female workers in the hospitality sector worker survey were mothers, and all but one were single-parents, mainly through male abandonment (see Chant and McIlwaine, 1995: Chapter 6). Nicole, a 24-year-old nightclub dancer, illustrates the dilemma facing women in the position of having to raise dependants alone. Having become pregnant at the age of 18 and turned to her boyfriend for help, the latter told Nicole that he no longer wished to have anything to do with her or their prospective child. Since Nicole herself was an only child whose parents had split up and left Cebu, she had nothing to fall back on but own devices. Although she tried to make a living by working as a promotions assistant for a dairy product company, the work was poorly paid and erratic, and the lure of higher earnings in the hospitality industry was too difficult to resist. Indeed Nicole declared that after all she had been through she had little else to lose by taking the step into entertainment work, and at least it had enabled her to fend for herself and her 5-year-old son.

While bar and nightclub workers do not receive a great deal more that the minimum wage of P105 for an average shift of seven hours (from 7 p.m. to 2 a.m.), most make extra money through commission on 'ladies drinks' purchased by clients during 'chat-up' sessions (a ladies drink is generally a diluted fruit juice for which an inflated sum of something like P150 [$6.25] is charged and of which 30 per cent goes to the girl herself). In addition, sleeping the night with a client may yield anything between P500 and P4000 ($20–170 US) (once the owner has received the bar fine women are entitled to negotiate their own price for sex and to pocket the entire sum). On top of this, many girls seem to form semi-permanent attachments with male clients, especially businessmen who visit Cebu on a regular basis. Returning clients who wish to see the same girl do not have to pay a bar fine on the second or subsequent occasion, but during the time they spend with her (sometimes up to one month), she receives no pay from her place of work and depends totally on the man in question. Many of the women stressed how well they were treated by older men or 'sugar daddies', who bought their children clothes and took them out for meals, day trips and so on. Some were being sent money to learn the languages of their regular clients, and one was actually being 'paid' to stay out of bar work by a former client, although the economic pressures of raising a small child made this impossible. For the men concerned, indulging the women and their families seems to mean little in the way of personal financial sacrifice, besides which the emotional and physical returns are regarded as highly favourable. Subscribing to widely held racist and gender stereotypes, foreign men tended to describe their Filipino companions as more 'affectionate', 'loving', and 'subservient' than women in their own countries, and one Canadian businessman went as far to say that he only 'bothered with women' on his trips to the Philippines since feminism in Canada had become a major problem and he had no wish to have girlfriends who were 'aggressive', 'authoritarian' and 'demanding' (Chant and McIlwaine, 1995: Chapter 6).

The household characteristics of women in the hospitality sector differed in various ways from those in tourism employment more generally. While the majority of female workers in hotels, shops and other non-hospitality establishments are single, childless women residing as daughters in their natal homes, this only applied to two of the fourteen female hospitality workers in our survey. Another two childless women lived alone (one rented a room in a boarding house, while the other lived on club premises), and nine out of the remaining ten respondents (all with children) were single-parents in the sense of living without male partners. Of these nine woman, three had formed independent lone-parent households; a further three resided with their children in their mothers' houses (in all cases the mothers themselves were also unpartnered on account of widowhood or abandonment); one woman rented a room in a relative's home, and the other two shared houses with female workmates. Two of these latter three women have fostered their children to parents in rural areas (in both cases to villages in the impoverished province of Leyte in the Eastern Visayas from whence they migrated). In fact, it is interesting to note that of the nine single women with children, as many as five were migrants to Cebu City, and one other had extensive migratory experience. This again is in direct contrast to workers in conventional tourism establishments who are likely to be native to the locality (see Chant and McIlwaine, 1995: Chapter 5).

There are two possible explanations for the comparatively high proportion of migrants among hospitality workers: one is that the earnings to be gleaned from sex work are generally far in excess of those in other occupations, especially in impoverished rural areas. In this way it is probable that hospitality employment exerts a greater drawing power to labour migrants from other parts of the Philippines. The other is that the anti-social nature of hospitality work means that it is less likely that girls native to the city and under the close surveillance of parents will be tempted, or even allowed, to work in sex bars. Indeed, as it is, the few natives working in Cebu's entertainment establishments tend to work as waitresses rather than dancers. The fact that everyone working in such establishments uses false names is indicative of the social opprobrium which tends to accompany the work. It is also significant that whereas migrants normally retain strong links with kin in areas of origin, this does not apply to sex workers. With the exception of the two migrant women who had fostered their children with parents in home villages, all the others had minimized contact, mainly for fear of bringing shame upon their families and of being upbraided for their lifestyles (indeed one of the fostering migrants said that she was known as the 'black sheep' of the family and, each time she went home, came under considerable pressure to give up her work). Another single parent, Arlene, who presently resides with her young son and one of her pregnant girlfriends, is so worried that her widowed father will find out what she does that she has only gone back to see him in Negros Oriental once in the past three years and has never invited him to Cebu. Having told him she is working as a cashier in a restaurant, she lives in fear that he will one day pay an unexpected visit and discover the reality of her circumstances (Chant and McIlwaine, 1995: Chapters 5 and 6) .

The fact that migrants away from their family contexts may feel freer to engage in hospitality employment, perhaps also explains the fact that the number of women with children living independently or with other girlfriends is large in comparison with figures for the locality in general. For example, census data for 1990 report only 14 per cent of households in Cebu City as headed by women, and in a detailed survey of 100 households carried out in one of the city's low-income neighbourhoods in 1993, only 17 per cent were found to be headed by women, and a mere 5 per cent to be independent mother–child units *per se* (see Chant and McIlwaine, 1995: Chapter 3). Part of the reason for low numbers of women living independently with their children is that lone mothers often face alienation and stigmatization from other people in the community: as such they may end up moving in with kin and becoming part of larger extended households as a means of either 'disguising' themselves or avoiding speculative or malicious gossip (*tsismis*) (when single mothers live with relatives there is less likelihood that they will lead what might otherwise be imagined to be a 'promiscuous' lifestyle) (see also Chant, forthcoming). At the same time, given that most employment opportunities for women are very poorly paid, it is difficult for lone women to raise their children without some kind of financial support from kin (ibid.). These economic pressures are, of course, less likely to apply to comparatively high-paid hospitality workers, and indeed where the latter are raising their children in their mothers' homes, they will not only often be the sole supporters of their own children but of the rest of the household as well.

Beyond the role played by economic solvency in accounting for female headship, the social ostracism faced by sex workers means that there is little to be lost from setting up independent and/or female-only households; as mentioned earlier, women living on their own are often suspected of earning their living immorally anyway so the additional cost is marginal. As it is, sex workers often seem to find that living without men results in the creation of more agreeable domestic environments. The absence of husbands and fathers reduces restrictions on women's behaviour, diminishes conflict and eradicates violence and, where women live with other women friends, co-workers and/or female kin, these benefits are enhanced by ready emotional support and practical help with child-care and domestic labour. Indeed, even if many sex workers recall the experience of male abandonment with anger or sadness, they often talk of the households that evolve around them as a refuge from their degrading, soul-destroying (and male-dominated) work environments in a way that women with partners tend not to do (see Chant and McIlwaine, 1995: Chapter 7).

Women's generally positive reactions to male-absent domestic environments are perhaps further borne out by the fact that many workers in hospitality establishments, even those without children, *stay* single, allthough there are other contributory factors. For example, one reason for remaining single is that it increases the chances of staying in work (employers are much less likely to want married women, and it is also rare that women will find spouses prepared to accept their involvement in the industry, even if sexual intercourse is not an integral part of their activities). Another reason for retaining single status is that, technically speaking, it enhances the prospects of marrying a foreigner. Around 50 per cent of women in the sample have aspirations of so doing, mainly because this would guarantee an income once their relatively short careers in entertainment work are over and might also provide a passport to international migration. Remaining single gives women the option to take up an offer on the spot if and when the opportunity arises. The fact that most are already mothers seems to have little bearing on their conjectured eligibility, with many claiming that long-term foreign boyfriends do not seem to mind spending time with their children (despite the fact that that they are not the real fathers) and, in fact, are often very indulgent with them. Indeed, one woman, presently engaged to a German, declared that her boyfriend had grown so fond of her 3-year-old son that this had been a decisive factor in his plans to move permanently to the Philippines to be with her. Somewhat surprisingly, perhaps, only two women in the sample had got pregnant, deliberately or otherwise, in the course of their work, and the seven single mothers with children by Filipino men had only entered the sex industry *after* having given birth, mainly because hospitality employment was the only sector offering wages high enough to survive alone. In this respect it appears that single-parenthood often pushes women into sex work, rather than the other way round, and pregnancy is not, as might be expected, a particularly common occupational hazard.

Having said this, other hazards of sex work include the ever-present threat of venereal disease, AIDS, or other physiological problems. Although the City Health Department provides free condoms and weekly check-ups for registered hospitality workers, condom-use is limited with the long-term clients who women regard as boyfriends.[29] Moreover, several women end up with fungal infections of the mouth or throat as a result of oral sex, and often face internal bruising and lesions as a result of aggressive and/or repeated intercourse. Hazards of a more social and/or psychological nature include the fact that most women realize that their prospects for continuing in this line of work are limited by age, and that it will be difficult for them to obtain comparably paid jobs in their 30s. Indeed, only two of the fourteen female respondents were 30 years or more. One, Salome, had an extremely youthful appearance and was hoping that her looks would last until she had paid her son's way through a private elementary education. The other, Alice, had been lucky enough to be taken on as a cashier/waitress once deemed by management to be too old to dance (see below). Aside from the limits imposed by their age, most women are also concerned to stop working in the sex industry by the time their childen are old enough to realize how they make their living. One 27-year-old hospitality worker with a son of 2 and a half years, for example, was dismayed to find that he had begun to refer to all the men she brought back to the house as 'Daddy'. Prospects for other employment, as noted above, are limited, especially in the formal sector where references are required. Here, women are caught in a double-bind. Providing references from previous workplaces exposes a woman's past, which in most cases is likely to put off prospective employers. On the other hand, covering-up previous employment makes it look as if women have little job experience, which, at the age of 30 plus, is also likely to lead to rejection. While some former dancers and hostesses might be able to continue working in clubs as cashiers and floor managers at later stages in their lives, these vacancies are relatively few in number. Thus most longer-term opportunities remain confined to the informal sector. The degree to which women will be able to set-up profitable own-account businesses may well, in turn, be limited by the cash and assets they are able to accumulate during their relatively brief spell in entertainment work: as noted earlier, earnings are high, but so, too, are women's outgoings, for costumes, make-up, beauty treatments and so on, quite apart from the routine expenditure incurred in raising children single-handedly. At the end of the day, therefore, even the economic gains from hospitality work provide little solution to long-term survival, and the majority of women face the prospect of returning to the poverty from whence they came (see Chant and McIlwaine, 1995; Chapter 6).[30]

Weighing up the position of women workers in tourism in Cebu, employment in hotels or other conventional establishments is likely to be less remunerative than in the entertainment sector, even if career stability (and indeed mobility) is probably greater. None the less, even in hotels, employers tend to prefer their female workers to be young and single, reflecting the pervasive recruitment of women on the grounds of physical beauty, especially for posts where 'natural charms' can be displayed to their best advantage. In this respect, the use of female sexuality is present in all types of tourism employment, and is simply a question of degree (see also Adkins, 1993, for an interesting discussion of similar patterns in tourism employment in the UK). However, despite the very negative ways in which tourism employers in Cebu (and in some cases in Boracay, as we shall see) exploit and commoditize femininity, one positive feature of hospitality work is that female employees are at least in the position, through relatively high earnings, to organize their lives in a manner different from that in mainstream society, particularly in respect of being able to raise their children alone and/or to establish household units which consist of friends and co-workers, rather than being subject to the rule of husbands or fathers in conventional patriarchal family structures. If this effective autonomy from men and prospective solidarity amongst women at the household level could be harnessed to develop greater political activity among women together with stronger demands for access to jobs and training, then there may be seeds from which to transform exploitation into advantage. Having said this, high earnings do not always translate into female headship, or even into much in the way of female power within male-headed households, as we go on to witness in the case of Boracay.

Boracay

While Boracay is one of the most important destinations for international visitors to the Philippines, tourism is of a much smaller scale than that in Cebu. Originally discovered by a foreign film crew in 1968, growth in Boracay has occurred through a mixture of foreign investment in medium-sized businesses and local 'backyard tourism' initiatives (Santa Maria, 1991). The island possesses a population of around 8,000 and has nearly 300 tourism establishments (hotels, shops and restaurants) with an accommodation capacity of around 1,500 rooms (many of which are actually small open-plan cottages which sleep up to four people). According to the Philippine Tourism Secretary (Vicente Carlos) and the Director of the National Economic and Development Authority (General Cielito Habito), Boracay is the centrepiece of tourism development in the country and reflects the twin strategies of the Medium Term Development Plan of the Philippines, namely global competitiveness and human development/people empowerment.[31] Unlike many other Philippine tourism destinations, Boracay is actively promoted as a 'family resort', with strict prohibitions on the opening of girlie bars and police discouragement of soliciting.[32,33] However, it is often the case that male foreign tourists meet women in either Manila or Cebu and then bring them to Boracay for periods of a week or so. Moreover, many local girls find foreign 'boyfriends' on the island who 'take care' of them for the length of their stay (see Chant and McIlwaine, 1995: Chapter 6). None the less, as opposed to the national picture where men are around three-quarters of foreign tourists, in Boracay men are only 55 per cent of visitors which undoubtedly reflects the lack of a formalized/above-board entertainment infrastructure on the island. In addition, the majority of tourists to Boracay are young, with around two-thirds aged between 15 and 35 years. Another deviation from the national picture (and Cebu), is the mix of geographical origins of foreign visitors to the island. Of around 15,000 foreigners who visited Boracay in 1991 West Europeans were predominant (70 per cent), with a further 11 per cent from the Middle East, 10 per cent from North America, 6 per cent from Australia, and only a handful from East Asia (DOT, 1991a: 104).

Most of the beaches in Boracay, unlike those in Cebu, are for public use, meaning that local people have access to them, not only for recreation, but also for work and, in this respect, there is considerable opportunity for people to create their own forms of livelihood rather than depend entirely on employers. This is important since, although educational prerequisites are not as important as in Cebu for work in the so-called 'formal sector' (hotels, restaurants, souvenir shops for example), for most types of self-employment such as beachfront-vending, motorbike taxi driving and boat transport, there is wider access for those with limited or no schooling.

In terms of the segmentation of male and female workers in Boracay's formal sector of employment it would appear that women have greater opportunity for work than in Cebu, and also that there is more fluidity in terms of men's and women's employment in different jobs. For example, out of a total of 226 employees in six hotels where interviews were held with owners or personnel managers, 95, or 42 per cent, were women.[34] This is a higher percentage than in Cebu (or indeed Puerto Vallarta) and, beyond this, women are found in a wider range of departments than in Cebu and in a wider variety of occupations.

Women not only predominate in housekeeping (averaging 86 per cent of the workforce in the six hotels in the survey), but are exclusively employed in laundrywork (although only three of the hotels were actually large enough to have separate laundry sections). As in Cebu, women also figure heavily in administration and accounts and in front desk duties, where they make-up around one-half and three-quarters of the workforce respectively. The only areas of hotel employment where women are regularly under-represented are gardening and maintenance, guest transportation (some of the larger hotels send guides in boats to pick up actual and potential guests from the ferry at Caticlan), security (most security guards are hired through agencies, as in Cebu), and to a lesser extent food and beverages. In the food and beverages industry women were on average only 24 per cent of employees and, as in Puerto Vallarta, the larger and more prestigious the establishment, the greater the likelihood that men will be employed as cooks and kitchen hands, and particularly as waiters, again because male food attendants are thought to present a more professional and stylish image (see Chant and McIlwaine, 1995: Chapter 5).

However, this last observation does not apply to restaurants independent of hotels on the island (out of four restaurants in which interviews were conducted, three are up-market establishments with some foreign involvement, and one is a family business). In these independent restaurants, women predominate in waiting at table, the rationale being in all cases that women will attract more custom (see Chant, 1993b). Much of this has to do with the nature of restaurants in Boracay which are, for the most part, open-plan and situated on the beachfront, where employees are required to stand outside and solicit clientèle. This is in direct contrast to hotels on the island, or indeed in Cebu, where restaurants are enclosed and do not rely on bringing in custom from public thoroughfares. The practice of using women to attract restaurant custom in Boracay tends to reinforce the common use of Filipino women's physical and social attributes as a means of stimulating business among a predominantly male clientèle (even where men are accompanied by wives or girlfriends, they are assumed to be the ones with money to spend). For similar reasons, virtually all employees in Boracay's tourist shops are female, the reasons cited including that female sales assistants attract custom and that they are more adept at arranging and displaying merchandise than men.

The predominance of women in commerce in the formal sector is also mirrored in the more independent/informal activity of ambulant vending whereby traders carry their produce with them and sell direct to tourists or to tourism establishments (see Chant, 1993b). The vast bulk of beachfront hawkers in Boracay are members of the Boracay Vendors and Peddlers Association.[35] As of 1993 the members of this organization numbered 247, of whom around 85 per cent were women (including illegal vendors the total number operating in Boracay is around 350). The kinds of items traded by vendors include services such as massages and manicures, and goods including T-shirts and shorts, 'native products' (mainly wickerware and shellcrafts), fruit, coconut oil, fish, light cooked snacks such as 'sticky rice' and boiled cassava, newspapers and ice creams. Exclusive areas of female activity include massages and manicures and the selling of fruit; women also predominate in the selling of T-shirts and shorts and Philippine handicrafts. Men, on the other hand, totally dominate the selling of fish, ice cream and newspapers. Fish selling excludes women because it is usually sold by the people who catch it and all fisherpeople on the island are male. Ice-cream retail is a male activity because considerable strength is needed to carry the heavy polystyrene containers which keep the products frozen. Finally, newspaper vending is a job which requires considerable mobility and an early start since newspapers have to be brought first thing in the morning from the nearest large town, Kalibo, which is over two hours away from Boracay by bus and boat (women are usually at home getting their children ready for school at this time). Beyond ambulant vending, two other types of tourism-related informal employment on Boracay are the ferrying of goods and people over the narrow stretch of water between Boracay and Caticlan on the mainland, and the motorbike and tricyle taxi services which transport provisions and passengers around the island. Both these activities, which have their own worker associations, are exclusive employers of men, reflecting in the case of boat cargo the traditional role of male Boracaynons as fisherman and seafarers and, in the case of the taxi service, the fact that transport in the Philippines is an overwhelmingly male domain.

Finally, home-based activities, some of which cater directly for the tourist market, provide the other main source of income on the island, particularly among women. Home-based enterprises range from individualized activities such as taking in laundry, to small manufacturing workshops which may engage the help of children (most workshops in Boracay are related to the shellcraft trade and involve people making jewellery, lampshades or door curtains for sale to wholesalers or souvenir shops), to home-based shops (*sari-sari* stores) or eateries/snack bars (*carenderias*).

Given a fairly wide range of employment opportunities for women in Boracay, it is interesting to note that different types of work tend to be associated with different groups of women. For example, in the formal tourism sector, most women workers are young (under 25) and single, whereas older married women with children predominate in the informal sphere of ambulant vending and home-based enterprises. Part of this distinction stems from working arrangements in formal establishments such as hotels and restaurants, where the vast bulk of employees (even those who are native to the island) are expected to reside on the premises as 'live-ins', usually sharing rooms with colleagues of the same sex. Payment for board and lodging is deducted from salaries at source and often provides a convenient way for employers to pay less than the legal minimum wage. Aside from the fact that formal sector employers generally desire a young workforce, for the reasons cited earlier, it is obviously easier to accommodate unmarried workers without dependents. As for women in the informal sector, a base on the island in terms of a home is usually a valuable asset in that houses can be turned over to economic use if the need arises.

In terms of the advantages accruing to women from tourism employment in Boracay, many stress how their work is generally interesting and sociable, and can sometimes be well-paid, especially in the high season. Indeed, one significant point is that there is often not much difference in earnings between the formal and informal sectors. The profits of ambulant vendors (especially masseuses), for example, and home-based female entrepreneurs are often greater than the wages (and tips) of employees in hotels, shops or restaurants. However, within the different sectors, men generally earn more than women. In formal employment, on the one hand, men (some of whom are married) make up a larger proportion of the workforce in the most prestigious hotels on the island which have the highest wages, the best tips and the fullest range of fringe benefits. Moreover, men are usually in better paid posts within hotels (see Chant and McIlwaine, 1995: Chapter 5). In the informal sector, male ambulant vendors tend not to have to work such long hours to earn the same as women, mainly because the goods they trade have a more ready market. This also applies to transport workers, who often turn down custom when people refuse to pay inflated rates for short journeys (Chant, 1993b). The fact that men appear to have the luxury to turn away business in a way that women cannot may well have to do with women often being the economic mainstay of households on the island, whereas men generally contribute little income (or time) to family life (Chant and McIlwaine, 1995: Chapter 3). Here there are some parallels with Puerto Vallarta where, because women are often in a position of being able to make reasonable earnings, men may withdraw financial contributions. However, while some Mexican women will leave their spouses if too much is taken for granted, those in Boracay tend to put up with these injustices to a greater extent *and*, in addition to tolerating husbands' 'vices', such as gambling, drinking, and even entertaining 'chicks' (other women), will frequently give them some of their own earnings to enable them to pursue these activities. Although Catholicism seems to be equally strong in both countries, reluctance among married women to separate on religious grounds seems to be reinforced by the legal prohibition of divorce in the Philippines, with the result that many end up enduring situations in which male inputs to household welfare amount only to the barest minimum (see Chant, 1995). The upshot of all this is that women are often heavily burdened with a dual role and little of their income translates into opportunities for personal advancement or autonomy. This also applies to some extent to young single women on the island, many of whom reside as 'live-ins' on their work premises. Most 'live-ins' are migrants from other parts of the Philippines, and in all but a few cases, remit an average of one-third of their wages to support parents and siblings in home areas (Chant and McIlwaine, 1995: Chapter 5).

CONCLUSIONS

In terms of what the findings of the above case studies mean for women's involvement in international tourism in a more general sense, the following issues stand out. One is that international tourism is not radically different from other economic sectors such as industry or agri-business, in that it comprises distinctively feminized segments which are usually towards the lower end of the occupational hierarchy in terms of status and earnings (see, for example, Sinclair, 1991). Where women do earn high sums of money (as in sex work), the social price is also high and the chance of maintaining their involvement in this activity in the long term is limited. Furthermore, expensive outgoings in the hospitality business erode women's capacity to save, especially where they are raising children on their own, as is usually the case. Another important issue is that female recruitment in formal sector enterprises catering for international tourists tends to draw heavily on male-constructed and male-biased gender stereotypes and to place women in occupations which in many respects crystallize and intensify their subordinate positions in society, whether through their assignation to low-level, behind-the-scenes domestic work as laundrywomen or chambermaids, or to jobs where their physical attributes are used to attract men or to gratify male sexual needs, as in front-line hotel, commercial and restaurant posts and in entertainment establishments (especially in the Philippines). A further cause for concern is that the profits from women's involvement in tourism labour usually accrue to men (and often foreign men) in their capacity as owners or shareholders of major tourism enterprises.

Despite these problems, there would seem to be some benefits for women as a result of growth in international tourism in Mexico and the Philippines. One is that in some contexts (particularly Boracay and, to a lesser extent, Puerto Vallarta) there would seem to be some scope for women to set up profitable own-account ventures, often using skills acquired in the formal sector. This is much less likely in industry (especially modern, export-processing industry) where women learn specialized, if simple, machine operations which have limited transferability to small-scale independent production units (Chant and McIlwaine, 1995: Chapter 7).

Another potential benefit for women workers in international travel destinations is their prospects for interacting with people from other countries. When this involves meeting other women (as is particularly the case in conventional sun-and-sea resorts like Puerto Vallarta and Boracay), it increases knowledge of gender roles and relations in other contexts and, combined with women's access to work and income, arguably leads them to be more reflective about their own situations. In Puerto Vallarta, for instance, exposure to North American tourists seems to have raised awareness that women have the capacity to control income, to take major decisions and to travel without their menfolk, and local women have often found this inspiring. In an alternative vein, even hospitality workers in Cebu are in the position of being able to formulate more rounded perceptions of men, in that coming into contact with a wide range of foreign males allows them to observe behaviour (married men indulging in sexual exploits behind their wives' backs, for instance), which gets them thinking about patriarchal institutions and practices more generally (Chant and McIlwaine, 1995: Chapter 5). Many of Cebu's sex workers, for example, comment frequently and openly on the injustice of women having to observe different laws to men within the context of wedlock.

A further (albeit double-edged) benefit for women is that tourism in both countries has created a situation where they have gained greater access to work (and often high-paid work) in the formal sector. This in turn contributes towards increasing women's visibility in national economies and forging some kind of public recognition of their roles in development. This has perhaps been especially marked in Mexico, where until relatively recently women had low rates of labour force participation and, as workers, were confined to predominantly informal activities such as domestic service (Chant, 1987, 1994b). Indeed Mexican women tend to equate paid work outside the home with having achieved greater freedom and control, and employment is usually regarded as a source of pride and power. In the Philippines, on the other hand, possibly because of long-term poverty and social expectations that women should find time to augment household income as well as to manage their domestic chores, many see employment as merely an additional chore (Chant, 1995). In some respects this could result from the type of work available to women in the country. In the case of sex work, for example, soul-destroying exploitation of their minds and bodies at the hands of male bosses and male clients means that women often have little sense of self-worth. To a lesser degree, the persistent emphasis on female ornamentalism in jobs within the conventional tourism sector can have the effect of undermining women's sense of personal achievement and professionalism. Beyond this, even where work itself is not especially exploitative or demeaning, the fact remains that women are usually the last to reap the returns from their labour in any personal or material sense within the context of the household.

While in Mexico and the Philippines alike, women's entry into the workforce is overwhelmingly motivated by, and oriented to, the needs of their families and their earnings are almost entirely dedicated to the immediate needs of dependents or other relatives, in the Philippines in particular, men's negligible contributions to household livelihood together with their tendency to appropriate wives' money for recreational pursuits means that women's employment often becomes more a tool of their subordination than emancipation (see also Chant and McIlwaine, 1995: Chapter 7; Santos and Lee, 1989: 38–9). The fact that the Philippine entertainment industry stands out as one of the few sectors where women can actually make a living adequate to raise children on their own, but that this is widely regarded as socially unacceptable, means that along with restrictions on divorce, many women remain trapped in conflictive and unsatisfying partnerships for fear of taking the step to sell their bodies and falling into disgrace in the eyes of wider society.

Having said this, hospitality employment at least provides earnings which allow women some measure of autonomy in terms of their household arrangements, in the sense of residing without men. This is also true of tourism employment in Puerto Vallarta where women workers seem to gain greater scope to determine their own lives and to eschew direct engagement with patriarchy at the domestic level. Even if women's work does not in itself enable (or even encourage) them to break-off inegalitarian relations with spouses, it at least allows them a margin of negotiation within the home environment. Indeed it is the intersection between earnings and control over domestic arrangements where the greatest gains of female involvement in tourism employment seem most apparent, especially when women head their own households. Not only are these women in a position of being able to control their lives to a much greater extent than when they live with men, but their daughters are also likely to gain from the resources apportioned by mothers, and by the role models they grow up with. Sons raised in these environments are also likely to be crucial actors in diminishing inequality in gender roles and relations in the future.

Although numerous institutional and societal changes are necessary if women are to use their domestic gains in any wider sense, the fact remains that, as a primary source of gender subordination, the household is a useful starting point of any major shifts in female status. With this in mind, efforts to enlarge and/or enhance women's foothold in international tourism employment should not only address such issues as female status, earnings and exploitation in the workplace, but give due support to initiatives aimed at improving women's position in the context of home and of society in general. The latter could include the more generalized provision of subsidized childcare, full entitlements to divorce, and the reduction of social sanctions on cohabitation and births outside wedlock, as well as access to abortion. Regrettably, these are low on the list of government policy agendas in both countries. Even in the Philippines, where the Development Plan for Women is calling for major changes in women's status and is encouraging state bodies to adopt measures to incorporate women's needs within such spheres as regional economic development and political representation, gender blindness and insensitivity to women's issues (together with the lack of effective tools for implementation and monitoring) means that improvements have been slow in coming (Chant and McIlwaine, 1995: Chapters 1 and 8). In the light of weak institutional commitment, much, at the end of the day, will depend on the strength of individual women, and, with any luck, their realization that greater strength is to be gained in numbers. In other words, movement from the bottom upwards is likely to be the most powerful (and feasible) instrument of change in women's lives. If feminization within tourism employment has any benefits, therefore, it is precisely in terms of bringing women together, not just as workers, but as women, who, given persistently discriminatory treatment by employers, by the state, and often by kin, neighbours and fellow citizens as well, may end up acting by themselves, for themselves, to demand fairer treatment in the workplace, the home, and in wider society.

NOTES

1 Fieldwork in Puerto Vallarta was carried out in 1986 and 1992 with funding provided by the Leverhulme Trust and the London School of Economics respectively. Fieldwork in Cebu and Boracay was conducted during 1993 under the auspices of a research grant for a project entitled 'Gender, Development and Poverty in the Philippine Visayas' from the Economic and Social Research Council (award no. R000234020). Preliminary fieldwork for the Philippine study in 1992 was financed by a series of small grants from the Nuffield Foundation, British Academy, Suntory-Toyota International Centre for Economics and Related Disciplines (STICERD), and the ESRC (award no. R000233291). The author gratefully acknowledges the funding received from these organizations, as well as the valuable assistance of the research officer on both the Philippines projects, Dr Cathy McIlwaine, and field assistants in the Philippines during 1993: Tessie Sato, Emma Galvez and Nonoy Gelito. The author would also like to extend thanks to Thea Sinclair for her penetrating comments on an earlier version of this chapter.

2 In both countries tourism is one of the top-ranking sources of foreign exchange earnings, being the third most important generator of foreign exchange in Mexico (EIU, 1991), and ranging between third and fourth in the Philippines (Republic of the Philippines et al., 1991; WRRC/PSC, 1990). During the 1970s, tourism was actually the largest source of foreign exchange in the Philippines, but in the wake of protests and bad press about sex tours in the early 1980s, especially those from Japan, tourism's relative importance as a dollar-generator has somewhat diminished (see Azarcon de la Cruz, 1985: 24–6; Eviota, 1992: 137; Matsui, 1991: 69–72; see also note 4).

3 South-East Asia is classified by the World Tourism Organisation as including Brunei, Indonesia, the People's Democratic Republic of Lao, Malaysia, Myanmar, Singapore, Thailand, Vietnam and the Philippines.

4 Although tourist arrivals to the Philippines fell further in 1991 in the wake of an attempted coup in 1990 in Manila and due to fears of Muslim unrest during the Gulf War, 1992 saw a substantial rise in numbers (EIU, 1992: 20). Moreover, between 1991 and 1996, the Department of Tourism plans to spend one billion Philippine pesos (c.$42,000 US) to revitalize the image of the Philippines and to renew tourism's role as a major dollar earner. This is deemed particularly necessary in the light of the withdrawal of US naval installations from Subic Bay (see *The*

Filipino 3: 1, Oct/Nov 1991 p.3 'Marketing Blitz Set to Woo More Tourists').

5 'Hospitality' establishments are officially designated as including nightclubs, dance halls, cabarets, cocktail lounges, massage parlours, steam and sauna baths, soda fountains, restaurants, beer houses and discothèques (see Perpiñan, 1983: 12; also Chant and McIlwaine, 1995: Chapter 6; NCRFW, 1989: 138).

6 Evidence for the continued availability and draw of sexual services in tourism to the Philippines is reflected in the fact that the male bias in tourist arrival composition has not declined since 1976 when 70.2 per cent of all tourists arriving for pleasure/holidays in the Philippines were male (see Mananzan, 1991: 106). The 1970s were the heyday of sex tourism in the Philippines, with President Ferdinand Marcos actively encouraging the activity as a means of generating much-needed foreign exchange (Raquisa, 1987: 218). In fact Eviota (1992: 137) claims that during the Marcos years, 'prostitution was not only allied with tourism, but did in fact support the industry'. Despite the current formal stand of the Department of Tourism against sex tours, the National Commission on the Role of Filipino Women (NCRFW) (1989: 67) notes that they still go on (see also Republic of the Philippines *et al.*, 1991: 142–3).

7 Pagsanjan, a scenic waterfall area in Luzon (Figure 6.2), is particularly noted for its child prostitution (see Fernandez-Magno, 1991 for further details on child prostitution there and elsewhere in the Philippines; see also HAIN, 1987; de Leon, 1991).

8 The publishing house in question was ICK booksellers and the publication *Southeast Asia for Men Travelling Alone* (see *Philippine Daily Inquirer* 4 April 1992 p.8, article entitled 'Japanese Feminists Hit Sex Tour Guide of Asia').

9 A Cebuana is a girl or woman native to Cebu.

10 Other brochures/leaflets on Cebu also make reference to women. For example the 1993 pamphlet published by the Department of Tourism in conjunction with the Cebu Chapter of the Women in Travel Association has an inset photo of a smiling girl on the cover and a section inside entitled 'night fun' which advertises clubs and bars with 'exciting floor shows and dancing'. The official Cebu and Bohol Traveller's Map also has an entertainment section divided into 'Day-time Pleasures' and 'Night-time Pleasures', the latter which also feature bars such as the 'After Six Supper Club', 'Bachelors Too', 'Silhouette Karaoke' and the 'St Moritz', all of which have semi-nude female entertainment and/or are contact spots for prostitutes.

11 For example, recent initiatives in Boracay include a major $23 million US dollar project to improve water supply, communications and telecommunications, sewerage and waste management funded by the Philippine and Australian governments (see NEDA Region VI, 1992)

12 Use of the term 'traditional' here relates to women's roles in the colonial and post-colonial periods'. In pre-Hispanic times, by contrast, women played a major part in generating the resources for household livelihood, being engaged in both farming and trading (see Blanc-Szanton,1990; Villariba, 1993: 7).

13 Penetrations of Catholic symbolism have probably been greater in Mexico than in the Philippines, partly due to the much more active colonization and settlement by Spaniards of the New World and partly due to the size and nature of indigenous populations. In her paper on the community of Estancia, Iloilo Province in the Western Visayas, Blanc-Szanton (1990: 352) notes that attributes of gender roles patterned on the Virgin Mary such as self-sacrifice, martyrdom, submergence of personal identity and so on are much less marked here than in Mexico. Moreover, pre-marital virginity, while important in the Philippines, is argued not to carry the same weight as in Latin societies (ibid.: 351).

14 Another important factor is that foreign travel is also seen to liberate people from 'traditional social obligations and norms which shape sexual conventions at home' (Abbott and Panos, 1992: 7) For detailed accounts of the causes and consequences of international sex tourism in South-East Asia in general see Graburn (1983), Hall (1992), Heyzer (1986: Chapter 4), Lee (1991), Sturdevant and Stoltzfus (eds) (1992) and Truong (1990).

15 Survey work in Puerto Vallarta in 1986 formed part of a larger project concerned with the analysis of female labour force participation and its interrelations with household structure, organization and survival among the poor in three cities with different types of economic base, the others being Querétaro, a modern manufacturing centre, and León, a traditional centre of shoe production. Fieldwork in Puerto Vallarta *per se* involved conducting questionnaire interviews with 92 low-income households, in-depth semi-structured discussions with a sub-sample of 24 respondents, and interviews with 21 employers selected from hotels, restaurants and the commercial sector (see Chant, 1991: Appendices 1 and 2 for full details). As noted earlier in the text, contact has been kept up with several households in low-income communities in each city, with ten in one Puerto Vallarta settlement (El Caloso) being re-interviewed in 1992 to provide an idea of changes occurring in household livelihood as a result of crisis and restructuring (see Chant, 1994b).

16 The figures for Puerto Vallarta and León relate to the household surveys carried out by the author in 1986 with 92 and 77 households respectively (see Note 15), and Querétaro in 1982–3 when 244 households were randomly sampled for interview. Household interviews did take place in Querétaro in 1986, but these were with a non-random sample of only 20 households (see Chant, 1991).

17 Interview with Mr Rene de los Santos, Director of Tourism Planning, Department of Tourism, Manila, March 1993.

18 Metro Cebu contains over 1 million people and consists of five cities: Cebu, Lapu-Lapu (Mactan), Mandaue, Toledo and Danao.

19 Most beach resorts forming part of Cebu's tourism hinterland are private and the hotels which own the land charge a 'walk-in' rate to those who wish to visit the beach for a day. The charge is generally upwards of P100 (c.$4 US – nearly one day's minimum wage) which means that many locals cannot avail of the facilities. This is recognized as a problem by the mayor of Lapu-Lapu City, Ernesto Weigel Jr, who in 1993 pledged 1 million pesos to supporting the development of two

public beaches at Ibo and Marigondon on Mactan Island (see *Sun Star Daily*, 15 April 1993, p.B2 'City of Sand and Surf').

20 Interview with Mr Alfonso Elvinia, Vice President of the Hotel, Restaurant and Resort Association – Cebu Chapter, Cebu City, March 1993. The HRRA-Cebu has been in existence since 1975 and had around 50 members in 1993. Criteria for membership include:

1 The establishment has to be in operation;
2 it has to be properly registered with the government and accredited by the Department of Tourism;
3 the business has to be 'respectable' and not engaged in 'highly questionable' activities. For example, the HRRA disapproves in principle of motels and 'quickie' hotel establishments.

It is perhaps surprising, given Clause 3, that several of the major hotels in town use photographs of young attractive women in their advertisements and boast of their 'charming and courteous frontliners'.

21 *Philippine Daily Enquirer* 16 Feb 1992 p.12 Article by Edmund Coronel 'Sex Tours Enjoy Cebu Revival'.

22 For example women working outside registered hospitality establishments, such as on the streets or in clandestine brothels, and who do not need health certificates as a condition of employment, are difficult for the authorities to trace and rarely avail of government health facilities for fear of exposure of themselves or their employers/pimps. An idea of underestimation from official figures comes from information on another tourist spot, Alaminos in Pangasinan province, Luzon, where only around 40 of the town's approximately 300 entertainers are reported to attend regularly for STD check-ups (see article 'A Town's Loss of Innocence' by Rina Jimenez David in *Philippine Daily Inquirer*, 15 April 1993, p.5).

23 The fieldwork on tourism in Cebu consisted of a range of formal interviews with employers and workers in the hotel, restaurant and hospitality sector, as well as discussions and/or informal interviews with other related groups such as male consumers of sexual services, union leaders, tour operators, women's groups, STD clinics and local tourism agencies such as the Department of Tourism Regional Office and the Cebu Chapter of the Hotel, Restaurant and Resort Association. Given the difficulties of gaining access to employers in the hospitality sector, interviews with employers were limited to four of the major hotels in the locality. As regards workers, interviews were held with sixteen hospitality employees and seven workers in 'conventional' tourism establishments (hotels and restaurants). A total of five tour operators were interviewed and ten consumers of sexual services. Additional further information on hospitality employment was derived from a survey of 100 households in a low-income settlement in Cebu City ('Rubberworld'). Out of these 100 households, five contained someone currently or previously engaged in entertainment-related activity (see Chant and McIlwaine, 1995).

24 Badger (1993: 3) notes that men predominate in the formal sector of the tourism industry in several developing countries.

25 A completed high school education in the Philippines is equivalent to 4–5 years of secondary school education in the UK, and a two-year Philippine college diploma is equivalent to 'A' levels. A college degree of three or more years is equivalent to one or more years of higher education in the UK (see Chant and McIlwaine, 1995: Chapter 3).

26 The Yakuza is a Japanese organization similar to the Mafia and has been particularly active since the Second World War. It is involved in prostitution, drugs and the control of labour (see Sturdevant and Stoltzfus, 1992: 337).

27 Foreign men often marry Filipino women as a means of setting-up business in the country. This is especially relevant to the hospitality sector where only 40 per cent foreign equity is normally permitted. Marriage to a Filipino woman allows foreigners full ownership and control (see Chant and McIlwaine, 1995: Chapter 6).

28 Although male sexual services are rarely on offer in girlie bars, Cebu's does have one or two 'greenhouses' (male brothels) which cater for homosexual demand (interview with Lihok Pilipina, Cebu City, February 1992) .

29 Mark Nichter's and Ilya Abellanosa's (1994) pilot research on commercial sex workers in Cebu revealed that condom use ranges from 40 per cent to 80 per cent with customers, and only 2 to 6 per cent with boyfriends or husbands.

30 This point is speculative since the fieldwork in Cebu did not comprise a targeted sample of former sex workers. Having said this, two of the five households interviewed in a settlement survey in Rubberworld (see note 23, p. 168) had former sex workers as members: one woman was a 34-year-old mother of three now reliant on renting-out rooms and occasional handouts from the fathers of the children; the other was a 23-year-old single mother living with her parents. The latter was being supported by a long-term Italian client except that her heavy addiction to *shabu* (a synthetic drug known in the Philippines as 'poor man's cocaine') had resulted in severe dissipation of funds.

31 See *Philippine Times Journal* 23 May 1993, p.11, article entitled 'Boracay: Centerpiece of Philippine Tourism'.

32 Interview with Edgar Decena, Coordinator, Boracay Island Tourism Administration, February 1992.

33 The principal police unit on Boracay Island is the Boracay detachment of the Philippine National Police (PNP). Attached to this is the Balikbayan Tourist Security Unit whose main objective is to protect the lives and property of local and foreign tourists. Together with the Island Tourism Adminstration (ITA, a dependency of the national Department of Tourism), these organizations work in a variety of ways to to prevent the development of a sex industry on the island. For example, any bar with displays of nudity and so on is immediately issued a writ by ITA either to close down or to 'clean up'. The ITA has also resisted instigating the practice of issuing 'health certificates' among the island's workers. While it is often compulsory for hotel, bar and

restaurant workers in other parts of the Philippines (especially places with large hospitality industries) to carry a card indicating freedom from 'social diseases', it is felt that certificates would be a dangerous first step towards acknowledging and legitimizing the operation of sex bars on the island. Other crime prevention strategies include police visibility, police patrols, and community relations activities: as far as possible the police try to maintain good relations with *barangay* (neighbourhood) captains, church leaders and so on as a means of pinpointing locals who might be getting involved in the generation of 'immoral earnings'. Having said this, prostitution does go on in Boracay and there are known spots including a discothèque and two bars where girls are available. However, operations are generally discreet and the police are reluctant to caution Filipino girls with foreign men in case these are 'normal' (genuine) boyfriend–girlfriend relationships. Morever, given the low incidence of money actually exchanging hands in public, scope for police intervention in individual cases remains limited (interview with Captain George Dadulo, Station Commander, PNP, Boracay, July 1993).

34 The fieldwork on tourism in Boracay, as in Cebu, consisted of a range of interviews with different employers, workers and related individuals/ organizations. Altogether a total of two shop owners were interviewed, four restaurant managers and six hotel/accommodation owners/managers. Included in the worker survey were four shop workers, four restaurant workers, eight hotel employees and fourteen ambulant vendors. In addition, information on tourism employment was gathered as part of a questionnaire survey with 60 low-income households in two settlements on the island (Balabag and Manoc-Manoc) and in-depth semi-structured interviews with ten of the households survey respondents. Contextual information was also gathered from the two tour operators on the island (7107 Tours and Swagman Travel), the two main business associations (BITZA/Boracay Island Tourism Association which represents foreign-owned establishments, and UBIBA/United Boracay Island Business Association), the Boracay Vendors and Peddlers Association (see note 35), the Boracay Multi-purpose Cooperative, the Island Tourism Administration, and the Philippine National Police. An attempt was also made to explore the attitudes towards sexual companionship with Filipino women of male visitors to Boracay by interviewing seven male tourists (see Chant and McIlwaine, 1995: Chapter 6).

35 The Boracay Vendors and Peddlers Association was set up in 1987 in response to the local office of the Department of Tourism's attempt to regulate commerce on the island. From this year onwards, vendors in Boracay have been required to gain an official trading permit and to become members of the association. In turn the association endeavours to regulate prices and also to control criminal activity (prior to the inauguration of the organization there was much petty theft among beach vendors). Initial registration in the organization requires a mayor's permit, clearance from one's *barangay* (neighbourhood) captain together with a residence certificate (although vendors do not have

to be resident on the island), police clearance, a health certificate, a joining fee and a licence to operate (in the case of masseuses for example). The cost of this package is in the region of P350 (c.$15 US), and is followed thereafter by annual licence renewal of c.P120 ($5 US) (Interview with Sally Casimero, President, Boracay Vendors and Peddlers Association, Manoc-Manoc, Boracay, July 1993).

REFERENCES

Abbott, Gary and Panos (1992) 'Along For the Ride: HIV and Sex Tourism', *WorldAids* 20: 5–8.
Adkins, Lisa (1993) 'Hors D'œuvres', *Tourism in Focus* 10 (Special issue on Women and Tourism Development): 6–7.
Aguilar, Delia (1988) *The Feminist Challenge: Initial Working Principles Towards Reconceptualising the Feminist Movement in the Philippines*, Manila: Asian Social Institute in cooperation with the World Association for Christian Communication.
Aguilar, Delia (1991) *Filipino Housewives Speak*, Manila: Rainfree Trading and Publishing Inc.
Aldana, Cornelia (1989) *A Contract for Underdevelopment: Subcontracting for Multinationals in the Philippine Semiconductor and Garment Industries*, Manila: IBON Databank Phils Inc.
Angeles, Leonora (1990) 'Women's Roles and Status in the Philippines: An Historical Perspective', in Marjorie Evasco, Aurora Javate de Dios and Flor Caagusan (eds) *Women's Springbook: Readings on Women and Society*, Quezon City: Fresam Press, 15–24.
Arias, Patricia (1990) 'Nueva Industrialización, Otros Trabajadores', *Ciudades* (Red Nacional de la Investigación Urbana) 7: 19–25.
Arizmendi, Fernando (1980) 'Familia, Organización Transicional, Estructura Social, Relación Objetal', in Carlos Corona Ibarra (ed.) *Antropocultura*, Guadalajara: Universidad de Guadalajara, 68–87.
Arizpe, Lourdes (1982) *Etnicismo, Migración y Cambio Económico*, México DF: El Colegio de México.
Azarcon de la Cruz, Pennie (1985) *Filipinas for Sale: An Alternative Philippine Report on Women and Tourism,* Quezon City: Philippine Women's Research Collective.
Badger, Anne (1993) 'Why Not Acknowledge Women?', *Tourism in Focus* 10 (Special issue on Women and Tourism Development): 2–3 & 5.
Barry, Tom (1992) *Mexico: A Country Guide,* Albuquerque: Inter-Hemispheric Education Resource Center.
Benería, Lourdes (1991) 'Structural Adjustment, the Labour Market and the Household: The Case of Mexico', in Guy Standing and Victor Tokman (eds) *Towards Social Adjustment: Labour Market Issues in Structural Adjustment*, Geneva: ILO, 161–83.
Benería, Lourdes and Roldan, Martha (1987) *The Crossroads of Class and Gender: Industrial Homework, Subcontracting and Household Dynamics in Mexico City*, Chicago: University of Chicago.
Blanc-Szanton, Cristina (1990) 'Collision of Cultures: Historical

Reformulations of Gender in the Lowland Visayas, Philippines', in Jane Atkinson and Sherry Errington (eds) *Power and Difference,* Stanford, California: Stanford University Press, 345–83.

Bridges, Julian (1980) 'The Mexican Family', in Man Singh Das and Clinton Jesser (eds) *The Family in Latin America,* New Delhi: Vikas, 195–334.

Brydon, Lynne and Chant, Sylvia (1993) *Women in the Third World: Gender Issues in Rural and Urban Areas,* (reprinted edition) Aldershot: Edward Elgar.

Bucoy, Rhodora (1992) 'Some Notes on the Status of Women in Cebu', *Review of Women's Studies* (University of the Philippines, Quezon City) 3,1: 33–50.

Bureau of Women and Minors (BWM) (1985) *Exploratory Survey of the Skills Training Needs of Rural Women in Selected Areas,* Manila: BWM, Ministry of Labour and Employment.

Castillo, Gelia (1991) 'Family and Household: The Microworld of the Filipino', in Department of Sociology-Anthropology (ed.) *SA21: Selected Readings,* Quezon City: Office of Research and Publications, Ateneo de Manila University, 244–6.

Chant, Sylvia (1985a) 'Family Formation and Female Roles in Querétaro, Mexico', *Bulletin of Latin American Research* 4, 1: 17–32.

—— (1985b) 'Single-parent Families: Choice or Constraint? The Formation of Female-headed Households in Mexican Shanty Towns', *Development and Change* 16: 635–56.

—— (1987) 'Family Structure and Female Labour in Querétaro, Mexico', in Janet Momsen and Janet Townsend (eds) *Geography of Gender in the Third World,* London: Hutchinson, 277–93.

—— (1991) *Women and Survival in Mexican Cities: Perspectives on Gender, Labour Markets and Low-income Households,* Manchester: Manchester University Press.

—— (1992) 'Tourism in Latin America: Perspectives from Mexico and Costa Rica', in David Harrison (ed.) *Tourism and the Less Developed Countries,* London: Belhaven, 85–101.

—— (1993a) 'Women's Work and Household Change in the 1980s', in Neil Harvey (ed.) *Mexico: Dilemmas of Transition,* London: Institute of Latin American Studies, University of London and British Acadmic Press, 318–54.

—— (1993b) 'Working Women in Boracay', *Tourism in Focus* 10 (Special issue on Women and Tourism Development): 8–9 & 17.

—— (1994a) 'Women and Poverty in Urban Latin America: Mexican and Costa Rican Experiences', in Fatima Meer (ed.) *Poverty in the 1990s: The Responses of Urban Women,* Paris: UNESCO/International Social Science Council, 87–115.

—— (1994b) 'Women, Work and Household Survival Strategies in Mexico, 1982–1992: Past Trends, Current Tendencies and Future Research', *Bulletin of Latin American Research* 13, 2: 203–33.

—— (forthcoming) 'Women's Roles in Recession and Economic Restructuring in Mexico and the Philippines', *Geoforum,* 23: 4.

Chant, Sylvia and McIlwaine, Cathy (1995) *Women of a Lesser Cost:*

Female Labour, Foreign Exchange and Philippine Development, London: Pluto.

Church, Timothy (1986) *Filipino Personality: A Review of Research and Writings*, Monograph Series no. 6, Manila: De la Salle University Press.

de Barbieri, Teresita (1982) 'Familia y Trabajo Doméstico', paper presented at the seminar 'Domestic Groups, Family and Society', El Colegio de México: México DF, 7–9 July 1982.

de Barbieri, Teresita and de Oliveira, Orlandina (1989) 'Reproducción de la Fuerza de Trabajo en América Latina: Algunas Hipótesis', in Martha Schteingart (ed.) *Las Ciudades Latinoamericanas en la Crisis*, México DF: Editorial Trillas, 19–29.

de la Cerna, Madrileña (1992) 'Women Empowering Women: The Cebu Experience', *Review of Women's Studies* (University of the Philippines, Quezon City) 3, 1: 51–66.

de Leon, Adul (1991) 'Economic, Political, Legal and Psychological Aspects: A Philippine Perspective', in Koron Srisang (ed.) *Caught in Modern Slavery: Tourism and Child Prostitution in Asia*, Bangkok: Ecumenical Coalition on Third World Development, 53–9.

de Oliveira, Orlandina (1990) 'Empleo Femenino en México en Tiempos de Recesión Económica: Tendencias Recientes', in DAWN/MUDAR (eds) *Mujer y Crisis: Respuestas Ante la Recesión*, Carácas: Editorial Nueva Sociedad, 31–54.

Department of Tourism (DOT) (1991a) *Boracay Island Tourism Development Project: Environmental Impact Statement*, Manila: DOT, Office of Tourism Development Planning.

—— (1991b) *Investment Opportunities in the Philippine Tourism Industry*, Manila: DOT.

—— (1992) *Visitor Arrivals to the Philippines, January–November 1992*, Manila: Tourism Research and Statistics Division, Office of Tourism Development Planning, DOT.

Economist Intelligence Unit (EIU) (1991) *Mexico: Country Profile 1990–1*, London: EIU.

—— (1992) *Philippines Country Report No. 4 1992*, London: EIU.

—— (1993) *Philippines Country Report, 4th Quarter 1993*, London: EIU.

Eviota, Elizabeth (1986) 'The Articulation of Gender and Class in the Philippines', in Eleanor Leacock and Helen Safa (eds) *Women's Work*, Massachussetts: Bergin and Garvey, 194–206.

—— (1988) 'Relations Between Women and Men', in SIBAT/CWR (eds) *A Development Framework for Women's Socio–economic Projects*, Manila: SIBAT, 46–8.

—— (1991) 'Sex as a Differentiating Variable in Work and Power Relations', in Department of Sociology-Anthropology (ed.) *SA21: Selected Readings,* Quezon City: Office of Research and Publications, Ateneo de Manila University, 157–69.

—— (1992) *The Political Economy of Gender: Women and the Sexual Division of Labour in the Philippines*, London: Zed.

Fernández-Kelly, María Patricia (1983) 'Mexican Border Industrialisation, Female Labour Force Participation and Migration', in June Nash and María Patricia Fernández-Kelly (eds) *Women, Men and the International*

Division of Labour, Albany, New York: State University of New York Press, 205–23.

Fernandez-Magno, Susan (1991) 'Child Prostitution: Image of a Decadent Society', in Sister Mary John Mananzan (ed.) *Essays on Women*, (revised edition) Manila: Institute of Women's Studies, St Scholastica's College, 129–43.

Francisco, Josefa (1990) 'Studies on Women Working and Living in Poverty', in Marjorie Evasco, Aurora Javate de Dios and Flor Caagusan (eds) *Women's Springbook: Readings on Women and Society*, Quezon City: Fresam Press, 25–33.

Francisco, Josefa and Carlos, Celia (1988) 'Women in Economic Crisis: A Study of Women's Condition and Work in Households of Selected Poverty Groups', mimeo, Women's Research and Resource Center, Maryknoll College: Quezon City.

Gabayet, Luisa and Lailson, Silvia (1990) 'Mundo Laboral, Mundo Doméstico: Obreras de la Industria Manufacturera de Guadalajara', *Estudios Sociológicos* VIII, 24: 547–70.

García, Brígida; Muñoz, Humberto and de Oliveira, Orlandina (1983) 'Family y Trabajo en México y Brasil', *Estudios Sociológicos* (El Colegio de México, México DF), 1, 3: 487–507.

García Colomé, Nora (1990) 'Mujeres Tejedoras de Zapatos en Comanjilla, Guanajuato', in Elia Ramírez Bautista and Hilda R. Dávila (eds) *Trabajo Femenino y Crisis en México*, México DF: Programa Interdisciplinario de Estudios sobre la Mujer, El Colegio de México, 53–77.

González de la Rocha, Mercedes (1988a) 'Economic Crisis, Domestic Reorganization and Women's Work in Guadalajara, Mexico', *Bulletin of Latin American Research* 7, 2: 207–23.

—— (1988b) 'De Por Qué las Mujeres Aguantan Golpes y Cuernos: Un Análisis de Hogares sin Varón en Guadalajara', in Luisa Gabayet, Patricia García, Mercedes González de la Rocha, Silvia Lailson and Agustín Escobar (eds) *Mujeres y Sociedad: Salario, Hogar y Acción Social en el Occidente de México*, Guadalajara El Colegio de Jalisco/ CIESAS del Occidente, 205–27.

González de la Rocha, Mercedes; Escobar, Agustín and Martínez Castellanos, María de la O. (1990) 'Estrategias versus Conflictos: Reflexiones para el Estudio del Grupo Doméstico en Epoca del Crisis', in Guillermo de la Peña, Juan Manuel Durán, Agustín Escobar and Javier García de Alba (eds) *Crisis, Conflicto y Sobrevivencia: Estudios Sobre la Sociedad Urbana en México,* Guadalajara: Universidad de Guadalajara and CIESAS, 351–67.

Graburn, Nelson (1983) 'Tourism and Prostitution', *Annals of Tourism Research* 10: 437–43.

Hall, C. Michael (1992) 'Sex Tourism in South-east Asia', in David Harrison (ed.) *Tourism and the Less Developed Countries*, London: Belhaven, 64–74.

Hart, Donn (1971) 'Philippine Rural–Urban Migration: A View from Caticugan, a Bisayan Village', in *Behaviour Science Notes* 6, 2: 103–47.

Health Action Information Network (HAIN) (1987) *Pom Pom: Child and Youth Prostitution in the Philippines*, Quezon City: HAIN.

Herzog, Lawrence (1990) 'Baja's Tourism Boom', *Hemisphere* (Summer 1990): 32–4.

Heyzer, Noeleen (1986) *Working Women in Southeast Asia: Development, Subordination and Emancipation,* Milton Keynes: Open University Press.

Hollnsteiner, Mary (1991a) 'The Wife', in Department of Sociology-Anthropology (ed.) *SA21: Selected Readings*, Quezon City: Office of Research and Publications, Ateneo de Manila University, 251–75.

—— (1991b) 'The Husband', in Department of Sociology-Anthropology (ed.) *SA21: Selected Readings*, Quezon City: Office of Research and Publications, Ateneo de Manila University, 276–84.

Iglesias, Norma (1985) *La Flor Más Bella de la Maquiladora: Historias de Vida de la Mujer Obrera en Tijuana, Baja California Norte*, México DF: SEP/CEFNOMEX.

Illo, Jeanne Frances (1989) 'Who Heads the Household? Women in Households in the Philippines', in Amaryllis Torres (ed.) *The Filipino Woman in Focus: A Handbook of Reading,* Bangkok: UNESCO, 245–66.

Institute of Labour and Manpower Studies (ILMS) (1984) *Women in TNCs: The Philippine Case – Are Women in TNCs Exploited?*, Manila: Department of Labour and Employment.

Institute for Social Studies and Action (ISSA) (1991) *Women's Health: Facts and Issues*, ISSA: Manila.

International Labour Organisation (ILO) (1993) *Yearbook of Labour Statistics 1993*, Geneva: ILO.

Israel-Sobritchea, Carolyn (1991) 'Gender Ideology and the Status of Women in a Philippine Rural Community', in Sister Mary John Mananzan (ed.) *Essays on Women* (revised edition), Manila: Institute of Women's Studies, St Scholastica's College, 90–103.

Javier, Carina (1991) 'The Queen of the South', *Cebu* (Department of Tourism Regional Office, Cebu City): 1, 43, 1–4.

Kennedy, Janet, Russin, Antoinette and Martínez, Amalfi (1978) 'The Impact of Tourism Development on Women: A Case Study of Ixtapa-Zihuatanejo, Mexico'. Draft report for Tourism Projects Department, Washington: World Bank.

King, Elizabeth and Domingo, Lita (1986) 'The Changing Status of Filipino Women Across Family Generations', *Philippine Population Journal* 2, 1–2: 1–31.

Lee, Pat (1981) 'Hotel and Restaurant Workers in the Philippines', mimeo, London: Philippine Resource Centre.

Lee, Wendy (1991) 'Prostitution and Tourism in South-East Asia', in Nanneke Redclift and M. Thea Sinclair (eds) *Working Women: International Perspectives on Gender and Labour Ideology,* London: Routledge, 79–103.

LeVine, Sarah (1993) (in collaboration with Clara Sunderland Correa) *Dolor y Alegría: Women and Social Change in Urban Mexico*, Wisconsin: University of Wisconsin Press.

Licuanan, Patricia (1991) 'A Situation Analysis of Women in the Philippines', in Jeanne Frances Illo (ed.) *Gender Analysis and Planning: The*

1990 IPC-CIDA Workshop, Quezon City: Institute of Philippine Culture, Ateneo de Manila University, 15–28.

Lomnitz, Larissa (1977) *Networks and Marginality: Life in a Mexican Shanty Town*, New York: Academic Press.

Long, Veronica (1993) 'Nature Tourism: Environmental Stress or Environmental Salvation?', in A.J. Veal, P. Jonson and G. Cushman (eds) *Leisure and Tourism: Social and Environmental Change*, Sydney/Ontario: Centre for Leisure and Tourism Studies, University of Technology/ World Leisure and Recreation Association, 615–23.

Mackie, Vera (1992) 'Japan and South-east Asia: The International Division of Labour and Leisure', in David Harrison (ed.) *Tourism and the Less Developed Countries*, London: Belhaven, 75–84.

Mananzan, Sister Mary John (1991) 'Sexual Exploitation of Women in a Third World Setting', in Sister Mary John Mananzan (ed.) *Essays on Women* (revised edition), Manila: Institute of Women's Studies, St Scholastica's College, 104–12.

Mangahas, Fe and Pasalo, Virginia (1994) 'Devising an Empowerment Paradigm for Women in the Philippines: The Importance of the Family in Urban Micro-enterprises', in Fatima Meer (ed.) *Poverty in the 1990s: The Responses of Urban Women*, Paris: UNESCO/International Social Science Council, 243–68.

Matsui, Yayori (1991) *Women's Asia*, London: Zed (2nd impression).

Medina, Belen (1991) *The Filipino Family: A Text with Selected Readings*, Quezon City: University of the Philippines Press.

Miralao, Virginia (1989) *State Policies and Women's Health and Reproductive Rights*, Women and Health Series No. 1, Manila: Institute for Social Studies and Action.

Moreno, Eugenia (1982) 'La Mujer y la Planificación Familiar', in PRI *Consulta Popular: Participación de la Mujer*, Mexico DF: PRI/IEPES, 32–3.

Moselina, Leopoldo (1981) 'Olongapo's R and R Industry: A Sociological Analayis of Institutionalised Prostitution', *Ang Makatao* (Asian Social Institute) 1, 1: 5–42.

Nagot, Maria Cristina (1991) 'Preliminary Investigation on Domestic Violence Against Women', in Sister Mary John Mananzan (ed.) *Essays on Women* (revised edition), Manila: Institute of Women's Studies, St Scholastica's College, 113–28.

National Commission on the Role of Filipino Women (NCRFW) (1989) *Philippine Development Plan for Women 1989–1992*, Manila: NCRFW.

NEDA (National Economic and Development Authority) (1990) Updates on the Medium-term Philippine Development Plan 1990–1992, Manila: NEDA.

—— (1991) *1990 Philippine Development Report*, Manila: NEDA.

NEDA Region VI (1992) *Boracay Services Infrastructure Project*, Iloilo City: NEDA Region VI Office.

NEDA Region VII (1992) *Profile of Central Visayas*, Cebu City: NEDA Region VII Office.

Nichter, Mark and Abellanosa, Ilya (1994) 'STD/AIDS Prevention and Prophylaxis in Cebu: Popular Beliefs and Practices Among Youth and

Commercial Sex Workers'. Research proposal, Department of Anthropology, University of Arzona, Tucson.
O'Grady, Ron (1983) 'Prostitution Tourism', in Peter Holden, Jurgen Horlemann and Georg Friedrich Pfafflin (eds) *Tourism Prostitution Development*, Bangkok: Ecumenical Coalition on Third World Tourism, 11–13.
Olofson, Harold and Cristosomo, Lorelie (1989) *Outsiders and Insiders: A Comparative Study of Socio-economic Benefits to Locals from Two Types of Beach Resort Development in Cebu*, Cebu: Area Research Training Center, University of San Carlos.
Perpiñan, Sister Mary Soledad (1983) 'Philippine Women in the Service and Entertainment Sector', mimeo, London: Philippine Resource Centre.
Pineda-Ofreneo, Rosalinda (1987) 'Women in the Electronics Industry in the Philippines', in Cecilia Ng (ed.) *Technology and Gender: Women's Work in Asia*, Diliman/Kuala Lumpur: Women's Studies Unit, University of the Philippines/Malaysia Social Science Association, 92–106.
PROCESS (1993) *Gender Needs Assessment in PROCESS-supported Areas in Panay, Bohol and Northern Luzon*, Iloilo City: PROCESS.
Raquisa, Tonette (1987) 'Prostitution: A Philippine Experience', in Miranda Davies (ed.) *Third World Second Sex 2*, London: Zed, 218–24.
Republic of the Philippines (1990) *Updated Central Visayas Regional Development Plan, 1990–1992*, Cebu: Regional Development Council, Central Visayas.
Republic of the Philippines with United Nations Development Programme (UNDP) and World Tourism Organization (WTO) (1991) *Tourism Master Plan for the Philippines*, Madrid: UNDP/WTO.
Reyes, Socorro (1992) 'Legislative Agenda on Women's Issues for the New Congress', *Lila: Asia Pacific Women's Studies Journal* (Institute of Women's Studies, St Scholasticas College, Manila) 2: 45–64.
Reynoso y Valle, A. and de Regt, J.P. (1979) 'Growing Pains: Planned Tourism Development in Ixtapa-Zihuatanejo', in Emanuel de Kadt (ed.) *Tourism: Passport to Development?*, Oxford University Press: Oxford, 113–34.
Rosario, Rosario del (1985) *Life on the Assembly Line: An Alternative Report on Women Industrial Workers*, Quezon City: Philippine Women's Research Collective.
Rubin-Kurtzman, Jane (1987) *The Socioeconomic Determinants of Fertility in Mexico: Changing Perspectives*, Monograph Series 23. San Diego: Center for US-Mexican Studies, University of California.
Safa, Helen (1981) 'Runaway Shops and Female Employment: The Search for Cheap Labour', *Signs: Journal of Women in Culture and Society* 7, 2: 418–33.
Sala-Boza, Astrid (1982) 'The Sitio Sta Ana Cebuana: A Sociocultural Study'. Thesis presented to the Faculty of the Graduate School, University of San Carlos, Cebu City.
Santa Maria, Felice (1991) 'The Ballad of Boracay', *Mabuhay* April 1991: 13–29.
Santos, Aida (1991) 'Do Women Really Hold Up Half the Sky? Notes on the Women's Movement in the Philippines', in Sister Mary John Man-

anzan (ed.) *Essays on Women* (revised edition), Manila: Institute of Women's Studies, St Scholastica's College, 36–51.

Santos, Aida and Lee, Lynn (1989) *The Debt Crisis: A Treadmill of Poverty for Filipino Women*, Quezon City: KALAYAAN.

Selby, Henry; Murphy, Arthur and Lorenzen, Stephen (1990) *The Mexican Urban Household: Organising for Self-Defence*, Austin: University of Texas Press.

Sevilla, Judy Carol (1989) 'The Filipino Woman and the Family', in Amaryllis Torres (ed.) *The Filipino Woman in Focus: A Handbook of Reading*, Bangkok: UNESCO.

Shimuzu, Hiromu (1991) 'Filipino Children in Family and Society: Growing-up in a Many People Environment', in Department of Sociology-Anthropology (ed.) *SA21: Selected Readings*, Quezon City: Office of Research and Publications, Ateneo de Manila University, 106–25.

Sinclair, M. Thea (1991) 'Women, Work and Skill: Economic Theories and Feminist Perspectives', in Nanneke Redclift and M. Thea Sinclair (eds) *Working Women: International Perspectives on Gender and Labour Ideology*, London and New York: Routledge, 1–24.

Sturdevant, Saundra Pollock and Stoltzfus, Brenda (eds) (1992) *Let the Good Times Roll: Prostitution and the US Military in Asia*, New York: The New Press.

Torres, Eduardo (1992) *Tiempo Compartido*, México DF: Universidad Autónoma Metropolitana, Unidad Azcapotzalco.

Torres, Eduardo (1994) 'Desarrollo Turístico, TLC y Cambio Social en la Frontera Sur de México: El Caso de Quintana Roo', *Anuario de Estudios Urbanos* (UNA-CAD, México DF) 1 (in press).

Truong, Thanh-Dam (1990) *Sex, Money and Morality: Prostitution and Tourism in South-East Asia*, London: Zed.

United Nations Development Programme (UNDP) (1992) *Human Development Report 1992*, New York/Oxford: UN/Oxford University Press.

University of the Philippines, Asian Institute of Tourism (UP AIT) (1990) *Study on Regional Travel in the Philippines 1990 vol. III*, Manila: Department of Tourism.

Villariba, Mariya (1993) *Canvasses of Women in the Philippines*, Women and Society International Reports no. 7, London: Change.

Whitam, Frederick *et al.* (1985) *Male Homosexuality in Four Societies: Brazil, Guatemala, the Philippines and the US*, New York: Praeger.

Wilke, Renate (1983) 'Gentle Women for Hard Currency', in Peter Holden, Jürgen Pfafflin and Friedrich Georg (eds) *Prostitution Tourism Development*, Bangkok: Ecumenical Coalition on Third World Tourism, 14–16.

Women's Research and Resource Center (WRRC) and Philippines Steering Committee (PSC) (1990) 'Towards a Preliminary Viewing of Child Prostitution and Tourism', *Flights* 4, 2: 4–6.

World Bank (1992) *World Development Report 1992*, Oxford: Oxford University Press.

World Tourism Organization (WTO) (1992a) *Yearbook of Tourism Statistics 1991 vol. 1*, Madrid: WTO.

World Tourism Organization (WTO) (1992b) *Yearbook of Tourism Statistics 1991 vol. 2*, Madrid: WTO: .

Young, Kate (1982) 'Population Growth and Motherhood: Who Controls Women's Fertility?', in Olivia Harris (ed.) *Latin American Women*, London: Minority Rights Group, 14–16.

Yu, Elena and Liu, William (1980) *Fertility and Kinship in the Philippines*, Paris: University of Nôtre Dame Press.

Zosa-Feranil, Imelda (1984) 'Female Employment and the Family: A Case Study of the Bataan Export Processing Zone', in Gavin Jones (ed.) *Women in the Urban and Industrial Labour Force: Southeast and East Asia*, Development Studies Center Monograph no. 33, Canberra: Australian National University, 387–403.

Chapter 7

Tourism and prostitution in Japan

Hisae Muroi and Naoko Sasaki

INTRODUCTION

In the Asian region, tourism has been promoted actively since the United Nations' declaration of 1967 as 'The Year of the Tourist'. Korea, for example, started to develop Chejudo, a small island off the south-west coast, as a resort in the early 1970s, the Philippines established its Department of Tourism in 1973 and Thailand set up the Tourism Authority of Thailand in 1979. The promotion of tourism also brought about a massive growth in female prostitution in the region. Since 1964, when overseas travel was liberalized in Japan, many package tours have been organized to popularize overseas trips among the Japanese. However, many package tours were marketed exclusively to men, particularly those to South-East Asian countries, which were promoted as a male paradise. Japanese male tourists' behaviour was severely criticized by such organizations as the Christian Women's Federation of Korea, which organized vigorous protests against sex tourism. These campaigns were subsequently internationally coordinated by feminists and pressure groups in South-East Asian countries, including Japan. The protest movements made a significant impact on Japanese Prime Minister Suzuki when he visited the ASEAN countries in 1981 and met massive demonstrations at the airport in each country. Japanese men started to hesitate about visiting these countries.

The result seems to have been a shift in prostitution which, while still widespread in tourist destination countries, is increasingly prevalent in tourist origin countries. Since the early 1980s, increasing numbers of women from South-East Asian countries have started to work in the leisure industry in Japan, mainly as bar hostesses, dancers and prostitutes. Those women working in Japan have experienced abuse and exploitation, physical coercion, threats, confinement and economic deprivation.

This chapter aims to analyse the effects of tourism on women from South-East Asia working in Japan. First, we will discuss the growth of tourism and prostitution in South-East Asia and the increase in Japanese tourism in these countries. The subsequent decline in Japanese sex tourism abroad and the background issues which persuade women to come to Japan will be considered in the context of the economic and social situations in both their countries and Japan. The 'double standard' which divides Japanese wives from women who work as prostitutes will be examined and we will show that there are also important differences between the Asian women who work in prostitution-related activities in Japan. Some of the Asian women's experiences in Japan and their responses to them will be discussed, based on interviews with them. Finally, we will consider some possible ways of improving these women's situations.

PROSTITUTION TOURISM IN SOUTH-EAST ASIA

The issue of prostitution and tourism has been discussed by a number of authors, for example, Awanohara (1975), Takazato (1983), Phongpaichit (1982), Truong (1983), Handley (1989), Lee (1991), Hiebert and Ladd (1993). Prostitution has, for a long time, been a means by which the governments of a range of developing countries have obtained increasing amounts of foreign income from relatively rich tourists from industrialized countries. The process by which the government of the Philippines instituted a policy of tourism promotion and expansion is discussed in several papers, and the conditions of the women who are employed in the sector are examined in Sylvia Chant's chapter in this book. Richter (1980, 1981) considered President Marcos' policies towards tourism, including the 1973 Presidential Decree for the Promotion of Tourism, and the ways in which the policies were formulated and implemented by his government. Wood (1981) describes the way in which loans from international organizations were spent on the construction of infrastructure for tourism as part of a strategy for achieving economic growth via tourism. However, these tourism-oriented policies generated large-scale prostitution.

It is not easy to identify when the first criticisms of sex tourism took place, since women's groups in both developing and industrialized countries have a history of campaigning to improve the status of prostitutes. Many of the authors who have been concerned with the issue have described conditions in the prostitution industry and the profiles of the women who work in it. ISIS (Inter-Cultural Studies Information Service, 1979) published a special edition on Tourism and Prostitution, focusing on the tourism industry in Asia and depicting the conditions in Korea, the Philippines and Thailand. Villariba (1993) tells of the situation of Filipino women and the forces which impel them to industrialized countries. The Ecumenical Coalition on Third World Tourism, a Bangkok-based organization, provides a wide range of information about tourism and prostitution, describing the background context and current situation, as well as proposing campaigns and measures against sex tourism; for example, Srisang *et al.* (1991) and O'Grady (1994) have highlighted the issue of child prostitution in Asia.

Besides the papers written by pressure groups, many academics have published articles and books on prostitution. Hall (1992) provides a review of prostitution in South-East Asia, examining Korea, the Philippines, Taiwan, Thailand, and Australia as a sex-tourist generating country. He concluded that sex tourism performs a function of commodifying people and that 'The sexual relationship between prostitute and client is a mirror image of the dependency of South-east Asian nations on the developed world' (1992: 74). In 'Thai girls and farang men', Cohen (1982) provides information about the short- and long-term relationships between prostitutes and tourists, based on interviews with Thai women, and shows how the economic gains made by the women are offset by significant social and psychological costs. Heyzer (1986) discussed the control of female sexuality as a local and international business, as well as the personal characteristics and contexts of the women and children who are involved in it. Academic arguments and empirical research were interrelated by Phongpaichit (1982), who obtained detailed information about the economic backgrounds of prostitutes during her meetings with them. Further analytical work on the economic aspects of prostitution in the tourism industry was undertaken by Truong (1983). It is the economic aspect of tourism which has been a major reason why the governments of South-East Asian countries have encouraged the growth of the sector, as will be discussed in the following section.

PROMOTING PROSTITUTION TOURISM

In Asian countries, tourism is an important means of earning foreign currency. In Korea, the government's plan to develop Chejudo, an island near to Japan, as a tourist resort aimed to attract 0.6 million tourists with the construction of hotels, casinos and kisaeng (prostitution) houses (Yamaguchi, 1980). In the case of the Philippines, from 1973 to 1980 tourists to the country increased by about 26 per cent and total foreign income from tourism reached $320 million in 1980. During this period, the government received large loans from such international organizations as the World Bank and Asian Development Bank for the construction of its tourism-related infrastructure, including luxury hotels and paved roads in sightseeing areas. One of the important advantages of tourism is that it creates jobs. However, as Wood (1981: 7) has pointed out, 'There is some evidence that hotels run by multinational corporations tend to generate less employment than locally-managed hotels', whereas 'the largest single such "spin-off" occupation is often left politely unmentioned: prostitution. It has been estimated that tourism has helped create 100,000 prostitutes in Manila alone.'

Matsui (1993a) claims that the governments of the South-East Asian countries increased their promotion of tourism to compensate for a decrease in exports in the late 1980s since, even in the first half of the decade, earnings from tourism sometimes exceeded those from the staple commodity, rice. The tourism campaigns of 'Visit Thailand Year' in 1987 stimulated a large increase in foreign tourists visiting the country. The number of Japanese travellers to the country rose from 108,500 in 1985 to 162,000 in 1987, a 49 per cent increase. Prostitution tourism in South-East Asian countries had, however, developed long before the 1980s. It is argued that prostitution spread over South-East Asia to provide the US army with relaxation and recreation after the Vietnam War broke out in the 1960s. O'Grady (1992) argues that the end of the Vietnam War, in 1975, left a huge prostitution industry in these countries, and describes how two types of prostitution occurred in Thailand: first, cheap prostitution for local people and, second, large-scale prostitution tourism. O'Grady (1981) also pointed out that many of the five-star hotels in Manila, which were built according to the Presidential Decree to promote tourism, were occupied by Japanese male tourists.

In the late 1970s and 1980s, many governments failed to act against sex tours because of the large amounts of profit generated by them. For example, even when Thailand was referred to as the 'brothel of Asia', high government officials introduced legislation which underpinned prostitution tourism (Mingmongkol, 1981). More recently, some high ranking officials have begun to question the promotion of tourism. Mechai Viravaidhya, Minister of Industry in Thailand, was the 'first minister to look not only at the financial benefits of tourism but also at its impact on the environment and society' (Kelly, 1991: 44) and proposed a 'Women Visit Thailand Year' campaign. Public statements by representatives of government and business have changed in the context of the many protests and criticisms which have been levelled at prostitution tours and in view of the spread of AIDS. The next section of this chapter will examine the changes in Japanese tourism to South-East Asian countries which have occurred in the light of such protests.

JAPANESE TOURISM AND PROSTITUTION

The 1960s – liberalization of travel abroad

Japanese prostitution tours to South-East Asia are said to have started in the 1960s, along with the 1964 liberalization of travel abroad and the growth of the country's economy (Japan Travel Bureau, 1991). Although travel abroad was just a dream for most Japanese and was initially limited to a few rich people, overseas travel approximately quadrupled between 1964 and 1970. Tourism was promoted in the form of package tours. 'JALPAK' tours, marketed by Japan Airlines, first appeared in 1965 and their all-inclusive nature and tour guides enabled lower income Japanese, with little knowledge of foreign languages, to travel abroad.

The numbers of Japanese travelling abroad were originally dominated by business tourists. In 1964, approximately 37,600 Japanese visited foreign countries for business purposes and just under 19,000 were holidaymakers. However, as early as 1965, for the first time, the number of tourists travelling abroad for vacations exceeded those taking business trips and the disparity continued to increase in subsequent years. During the 1960s, Japanese tourists tended to travel to geographically proximate countries, particularly Taiwan and Korea, as is shown in Table 7.1, and the numbers of Japanese visiting these countries, as well as the Philippines and Thailand, increased considerably during the latter part of the decade. It has

Table 7.1   Geographically proximate destinations of Japanese tourists

	Taiwan	Korea	Philippines	Thailand
1964	5,225	1,846	2,391	3,399
1967	40,357	19,213	6,134	7,857
1969	100,927	31,111	8,086	12,948
1970	113,676	45,269	7,204	12,946
1973	341,096	411,189	30,072	68,195
1975	358,621	319,984	119,876	69,890
1977	482,832	447,519	145,689	79,090
1979	618,538	526,327	190,637	89,140
1980	584,641	428,008	187,445	93,413
1983	572,898	407,335	143,934	100,327
1985	618,511	480,583	136,513	108,460
1987	806,487	707,906	134,204	161,955

Source: Annual Report of Statistics on Legal Migrants, Ministry of Justice, 1965–88

been argued that the main beneficiaries of this boom were middle-aged men, many of whom were participating in prostitution tours.

The 1970s – Japanese tourists to South-East Asia

During the 1970s, the numbers of Japanese tourists continued to increase greatly (see Table 7.1) and the main destinations were countries within the South-East Asia region. Arrivals were dominated by men, who constituted 80–90 per cent of all travellers from Japan in 1979, in contrast to tourism to West European countries and the USA, where men were 50–60 per cent of the total, as is clear from Table 7.2.

In the case of Korea, for example, the number of tourists from Japan rose from just over 45,000 in 1970 to over 411,000 in 1973 and to over 526,000 in 1979, over 90 per cent of whom were men. Many men visited the newly developed resort of Chejudo, whose kisaeng tours had become well-known after their promotion by the mass media (Kishimoto, 1984). One subsidiary of a large-scale car manufacturing company was reported to provide overseas trips for workers who made high profits for the firm, the destinations always being countries in the South-East Asia region, including Korea, Taiwan and Thailand. 'Mr Ogawa', who joined a tour as a reward for his sales profit, described how he bought a girl in Thailand and how, another time, three Japanese men from the same company

Table 7.2   Destinations of Japanese tourists by sex, 1979

Country	Total	Male	Female	Male as % of total
US	1,410,320	837,504	572,816	59.4
Taiwan	618,538	565,223	53,315	91.4
Korea	526,327	493,100	33,227	93.7
Hong Kong	392,746	256,814	135,932	65.4
Philippines	190,637	159,522	31,115	83.7
France	166,622	84,162	82,460	50.5
Singapore	106,403	71,014	35,389	66.7
UK	97,295	57,659	39,636	59.3
Thailand	89,140	70,304	18,836	78.9
Indonesia	57,406	44,373	13,033	77.3
West Germany	47,109	34,277	11,832	74.3
Others	336,755	241,440	95,315	71.7
Total	4,038,298	2,915,392	1,122,906	72.2

Source: *Annual Report of Statistics on Legal Migrants*, Ministry of Justice, 1980

brought Thai girls (prostitutes) to their hotel in Bangkok. It was argued that:

> this company has been making use of sex tours as a reward to sales workers for more than ten years. . . . Although they do not attract them as before, since workers have got used to them and their wives are against them, the company cannot find better rewards than giving an opportunity to go on sex tours.
>
> (Tomioka, 1990: 26–27)

However, he also mentioned that the company's policy has been changing in recent years.

The 1980s – the era of the '*Japayuki-san*'

Following the boom of the 1970s, the structure of Japanese prostitution tourism changed in the 1980s. From 1980 to 1987, there was lower growth in the numbers of men travelling to Korea, the Philippines, Taiwan and Thailand. Traditionally, the number of men who were tourists had exceeded the number of women, but from 1981 onwards, the rate of growth in the number of Japanese women who travelled to most of the countries exceeded that for men, as is indicated by Table 7.3. Women became the object of increasing attention from the viewpoint of marketing tourism. In

Table 7.3 Japanese tourists' destinations by sex, 1980–87

	Taiwan		Korea		Philippines		Thailand	
	Male	Female	Male	Female	Male	Female	Male	Female
1980	524,526	60,115	400,321	27,687	154,481	32,964	72,610	20,803
1983	481,087	91,811	364,973	42,362	111,716	32,218	74,652	25,675
1985	501,662	116,849	417,429	63,154	103,596	32,917	79,466	28,994
1987	631,249	175,238	593,652	114,254	103,236	27,968	113,450	48,505

Source: Annual Report of Statistics on Legal Migrants, Ministry of Justice, 1981–88

1987, the JALPAK 'AVA' cheap tour was produced, targeted at young women office workers. The company also introduced a female marketing group, 'VIE', to collect information about women's needs in tourism, which were reflected in product planning by women involved in tourism marketing.

As the growth in the number of male tourists to South-East Asian countries declined during the 1980s and that of Japanese women tourists increased, the number of women coming to Japan from South-East Asia rose dramatically. Data for the number of migrants entering Japan from Taiwan, Korea, the Philippines and Thailand are given in Table 7.4. The figures for Koreans and Taiwanese are relatively high, as they have a long history of living in Japan. In the case of Thai immigrants between the ages of 15 and 24 years, the numbers of women exceed those of men. The data for Filipinos demonstrate that, between the ages of 15 and 29, there are considerably more women immigrants than men and, in 1982, the numbers of women were almost eight times those of men. Most of these women received entertainer visas to work in Japan and the number of '*Japayuki-san*' – foreign girls coming to Japan to work as prostitutes – increased dramatically.

The background to the increase in immigration into Japan by girls and women from South-East Asia is one of resistance to sex tourism. In 1972, for example, the Christian Women's Federation of Korea formulated and publicized a declaration opposing sex tours and, in 1973, university students of Korea organized a large demonstration, at Kimpo Airport, against Japanese coming on kisaeng tours. Women's groups in Japan also organized a demonstration at Haneda Airport in 1974. These demonstrations are argued to be one reason why tourism by male Japanese shifted from Korea to South-East Asian countries, where sex tours flourished in the late 1970s and early 1980s. However, the protest campaigns also spread to the Philippines and Thailand and male tourists from Japan subsequently met criticisms and protests throughout South-East Asia. Within the month of January 1981, when Prime Minister Suzuki paid an official visit to the ASEAN countries, *Asahi Shimbun*, one of the leading newspapers in Japan, published a range of articles which reported on the protest movement against sex tours to these countries. Many demonstrations and meetings were organized and letters and declarations of protest were sent to Prime Minister Suzuki.

A number of protests by Filipino women took place in Manila and were coordinated with action by Japanese women (Matsui, 1991).

Table 7.4 Migration into Japan by age and sex, 1982–92

Year	Age	Taiwan Men	Taiwan Women	Korea Men	Korea Women	Philippines Men	Philippines Women	Thailand Men	Thailand Women
	Total	311125		284598		37873		31422	
	All ages	142116	169009	183831	100767	15389	22489	16959	14463
1982	15–19	840	4086	2273	2107	466	1482	488	588
	20–24	2990	17937	4743	7882	1455	7826	1643	2093
	25–29	14274	28198	13019	11175	2443	5181	3006	2804
	Total	331634		283971		47887		43940	
	All ages	155341	176293	188381	95590	17357	30530	23846	20094
1983	15–19	1202	4562	2401	2016	695	1904	723	878
	20–24	3538	17908	4868	8596	1487	10502	2208	2670
	25–29	15853	29472	14267	11496	2409	7012	4009	3847
	Total	351294		292483		49511		45978	
	All ages	166765	184529	192285	100198	16062	33449	24909	21069
1984	15–19	1143	4199	2292	2208	557	2438	812	827
	20–24	3467	17912	5461	9630	1400	13496	2284	2785
	25–29	16336	29413	15674	13168	2481	7428	4199	4037
	Total	356934		296708		65529		44123	
	All ages	167651	189238	201342	95366	21106	44423	24749	19374
1985	15–19	1332	5101	2897	2799	1012	3002	776	748
	20–24	3465	18368	6036	8559	2197	17664	2175	2210
	25–29	14927	28415	16842	11532	3152	9376	4095	3619
	Total	300272		299602		80508		30296	
	All ages	145786	154486	199617	99985	22058	58450	17452	12844
1986	15–19	1068	4468	2528	2569	697	6651	515	494
	20–24	3517	16631	5336	8052	2934	28231	1613	1685
	25–29	14606	25180	17612	12941	4388	11966	2972	2684
	Total	360636		360159		85267		33719	
	All ages	174979	185657	230256	129903	21395	63872	19479	14240
1987	15–19	1260	5403	2891	3453	647	7818	473	783
	20–24	4498	20840	6155	9731	2604	30118	2039	2514
	25–29	18305	29160	21494	15662	4141	13516	3219	2849

Table 7.4   continued

Year	Age	Taiwan Men	Taiwan Women	Korea Men	Korea Women	Philippines Men	Philippines Women	Thailand Men	Thailand Women
	Total	392723		515806		86567		41994	
	All ages	189468	203255	325320	190487	18881	67686	22797	19197
1988	15–19	1495	6138	3927	4856	601	6395	513	1462
	20–24	5198	22984	9458	14393	2546	34005	2877	4873
	25–29	22008	33580	31919	21642	3127	14311	4086	4095
	Total	501907		806065		88296		49117	
	All ages	230953	270954	497974	308091	21437	66859	28180	20937
1989	15–19	2237	8157	6119	8070	610	4410	730	1145
	20–24	6736	29355	18294	30674	2884	30986	3300	3882
	25–29	26287	41283	61130	42812	3407	15314	5203	4255
	Total	610652		978984		108292		69477	
	All ages	272124	338528	585797	393187	24956	83336	38109	31368
1990	15–19	2642	10861	6880	10192	765	3917	1048	1607
	20–24	9114	36137	24928	42366	3659	37920	4359	5195
	25–29	30808	50530	76044	56297	4191	20521	6914	6190
	Total	686076		1097601		125329		105666	
	All ages	306158	379918	632619	464982	25619	99710	58200	47466
1991	15–19	3569	11657	7196	10964	711	7114	1595	2527
	20–24	10253	39132	28143	57176	4293	43690	7690	10020
	25–29	33992	55023	81937	66210	4793	25380	11409	10639
	Total	745835		1094724		120660		97568	
	All ages	331413	414422	602572	492152	24686	95974	52094	45474
1992	15–19	3479	12692	7504	10662	537	2291	1549	1204
	20–24	11027	40498	24862	59379	3793	38029	6347	8244
	25–29	36052	57990	72959	70094	4773	29778	9659	9601

Source: Annual Report of Statistics on Legal Migrants, Ministry of Justice, 1981–93
Note: * The number includes that of re-entrants.

On 5 January 1981, five women, representing fifty organizations which were involved in matters relating to women, religion, health and race, held a news conference and read out a letter addressed to Suzuki, protesting against sex tours by Japanese men. Newspapers from the two countries took up the topic and published articles criticizing Japan. Sixteen groups organized a forum to protest against Japanese prostitution tours in Asia and received messages of support from Japanese women's groups. In the same period, *Asahi Shimbun* reported that a human rights group was planning protest actions in Bangkok, and the newspaper *Thai Rat* stated its appreciation for the movement in Manila. The paper also reported that five women's groups from the national University, the 'Friends of Women' group and seven organizations involved in issues concerned with women and religion, had sent letters of protest to the deputy prime minister of Thailand and Prime Minister Suzuki. On the same day, a demonstration was organized by Thai people in front of the Japanese Embassy in Bangkok.

These actions put effective pressure on the government of Japan and, in the same month, the Department of Tourism of the Ministry of Transportation in Japan took action against a travel agency which had organized prostitution tours. The criticisms and protests which had greeted Japanese male tourists during the 1970s and 1980s had the effect of decreasing the numbers of sex tours to South-East Asia and, instead, women from the region started to come to Japan.

MIGRANT WORKERS

People migrate for various reasons. Migrant workers abroad aim to earn foreign currency, of which a large proportion is remitted to their countries of origin. Migration also increases employment opportunities for the people who remain in the country. In addition, ex-migrant workers can transfer technologies from more industrialized countries. It has been pointed out that more women migrate for economic reasons than for individual or social motives (United Nations Population Fund, 1993: 25):

> Although women are often thought of as 'passive movers', migrating only to join or follow family members, research has found that economic rather than personal or social considerations predominate.

The United Nations Population Fund also refers to Findley and Williams' (1991) finding that 50–70 per cent of migrant women in South-East Asia, Latin America and the Caribbean move to search for jobs. In Latin America, the Philippines and the South Pacific, young women migrate to aid their families and send money to their families more often than men, although their earnings are usually lower.

Various reports and articles about women from South-East Asia support Findley and Williams' findings. Miyoshi (1986), for example, cites a girl from Davao who came to Manila to earn money to send to her family. She also refers to the fact that 70 per cent of girls and women working in the hospitality sector in Manila are elder sisters. Ogawa (1985) explains how *japayuki-san* at a city in Shikoku Island came to Japan for the sake of their families. The rest of this section discusses the economic reasons why Asian women work as prostitutes.

The size of the economy: urban and rural areas in Thailand

Migrant workers from rural areas usually enter urban areas of their own country before moving to richer countries. People move to the places where they hope to get jobs. Taking the example of Thailand, the huge difference in economic wealth between urban and rural areas is often described as the reason for migrating. In 1988, the economic structures of the three regions of the north-east, north and south differed considerably from that of Bangkok, as is indicated by Table 7.5. The agricultural sector accounted for between 32 per cent and 37 per cent of gross domestic product in the three regions while, in Bangkok, it was only 3 per cent compared with the 47 per cent and 50 per cent shares of industry and services respectively. There was a considerable gap between the economic wealth of Bangkok and that of the remaining regions, with the exception of the Central region; while 16 per cent of the total population of Thailand resided in Bangkok, it accounted for half of total gross domestic product.

It is clear that workers migrate to urban areas to look for better lives. Phongpaichit (1982), for example, explained how, although the ratio of earnings outside Bangkok to those in the city increased during the 1960s and 1970s, earnings in Bangkok remained considerably greater than those in the other regions, as is shown in Table 7.6. It is clear that Bangkok has grown in economic terms, leaving the other regions behind, and this induces people to migrate from rural areas in search of a better standard of living.

This does not explain why many girls chose prostitution as their jobs. Examination of monthly pay by different occupations at the end of the 1970s, given in Table 7.7, shows at least one of the reasons; compared with other jobs, women who work as prostitutes

Table 7.5 Gross domestic product by region: Thailand (1988, current prices, millions of baht)

	North-east	North	South	Central	Bangkok	Total
Agriculture	57,281	58,733	53,387	57,325	23,600	250,384
Industry	36,556	39,477	23,889	86,362	353,805	540,089
Services	85,663	73,529	68,920	111,145	377,248	716,504
Total GDP	179,500	171,796	146,196	254,833	754,651	1,506,977
Percentage	12	11	10	17	50	100
Population						
Percentage	35	19	13	17	16	100

Source: National Income of Thailand, Office of the National Economic and Social Development Board (1990)

Table 7.6 Family earnings by region relative to earnings in Bangkok

	1962–63	1968–69	1975–76
North-east	32	29	44
North	32	32	44
South	50	34	53
Central	52	48	66
Bangkok	100	100	100

Source: *Income Consumption and Poverty in Thailand 1962–63 to 1975–76*,
IBRD, p. 20, cited in Phongpaichit (1982: 28)
Note: Earnings in Bangkok are considered as 100

or masseuses gain far higher earnings. This is a major factor
inducing girls to move from their local area to work in the urban
service sector, including the tourism industry.

Many people migrate to obtain jobs and to support their families.
They also migrate to earn more money to purchase consumer goods.
The change of lifestyle in Thai villages is considered by Takigawa
(1985), who describes the changes brought about by the introduction
of a money economy. People who used to weave their clothes at
home now buy goods made in factories. The commercialization of
products by the mass media, and the spread of a credit system, lead
to an increase in expenditure by farmers and causes the migration of
village people to the urban area in search of jobs. Women work as
prostitutes in order to obtain money, for motives ranging from the
desire to help their families to survive in conditions of extreme
poverty, to gaining additional earnings for spending on commercial
products.

Table 7.7 Monthly pay by occupation in Thailand, 1982

Occupation	Monthly Pay (baht)
Housemaid	150–450
Waitress	200–500
Construction labourer	200–500
Factory worker	200–500
Beauty Salon	400–600
Clerical Worker	600–1000
Service worker	800–1500
Prostitute or masseuse	10,000 + bonus

Source: Phongpaichit, (1982: 8)

Size of economy: Japan and South-East Asia

The value of gross national product (GNP) can be used as a measure of the differences in wealth between countries. The economic power of Japan far exceeds that of other South-East Asian countries, as is illustrated in Table 7.8. Even Korea, which is counted as one of the newly industrialized economies (NIEs), and which accomplished dramatic growth during the 1980s, is still far behind Japan; in 1991, for example, the per capita GNP of Japan was about four times greater than that of Korea.

Although Thailand also grew rapidly in the late 1980s, its GNP is small compared with that of Japan and that of the Philippines is even lower. People migrate for the purpose of getting jobs and money, and migration between Japan and the South-East Asian countries is argued to be due to the economic imbalance between them. However, migration is also caused by circumstances specific to different individuals, as is illustrated by the motives which three Thai women gave for working in Japan (Tezuka, 1992: 109):

A) 'I wanted to renovate a house for my child, as we lived in a miserable house which might fall down just because of a strong wind.'

B) 'We needed money as my father was sick. My mother could not work in farming as she had a problem with her waist. I decided to come to Japan as a debt only kept on increasing.'

C) 'I just wanted to be free from a poor life in a house with no toilet and kitchen. I also wanted to get electrical appliances.'

Table 7.8   Gross national product per capita (US$)

Year	Japan	Korea	Philippines	Thailand
1971	2,130	310	240	210
1980	9,890	1,520	690	670
1991	26,930	6,330	730	1,570

Source: World Bank (1973, 1982, 1993)

NATIONAL POLICY: SENDING WORKERS ABROAD

The Philippines

The Philippines has a history of sending workers abroad. The Statistics Office of the Republic of the Philippines (1989: 660) says that, 'There are two mainstreams of manpower outflow; first is permanent migration, wherein the workers leave on a more or less permanent basis; the second, contract or temporary migration.'

It describes how the first category of migration started in the early 1900s. After the USA took over the country as a colony, the country sent about 110,000 workers to Hawaii to provide cheap labour for pineapple plantations. The second category of migrant labour commenced after World War II, when the country sent many labourers to American strongholds to work on the rehabilitation and reconstruction of these areas. From the end of the 1960s to the early 1970s, many doctors and nurses were employed abroad. When the Middle East was enjoying a construction boom, a large number of Filipinos went to work in Arab countries.

In 1974, the government of the Philippines organized the Overseas Employment Development Board and, in 1982, it established the Philippines Overseas Employment Agency to help Filipinos to work abroad. The Philippines National Statistics Office estimates that workers remitted a total of $856.8 million in foreign earnings in 1988, equal to about 10 per cent of the country's export earnings in that year. In 1993, approximately $2.5 billion was sent to the country by migrant workers, through the national bank. The total amount, when remittances via private channels are included, was around four times greater, accounting for just under 20 per cent of the country's GDP in the same year.

During the 1980s, the majority of Filipinos who worked abroad were employed in the construction sector. However, the number of workers in the service sector, in which many women were employed, increased considerably during the decade and just exceeded the number of production process, transport workers and labourers in 1987. Many women worked as maids in Hong Kong and Europe and some were employed as teachers in Africa (Utsumi and Matsui, 1988). While 13,400 Filipinos were employed as 'entertainers' overseas in 1982, by 1987 the number had risen dramatically, to just under 40,000. This increase appears to be related to the decrease in the number of Japanese tourists to the

Philippines in the 1980s, along with the protests against prostitution tourism in the country. In 1988, President Aquino's government announced that the country was to stop sending Filipino maids to foreign countries (Sasaki, 1991) because of the vulnerable situations in which many found themselves and stated that the controls would only be removed for host countries which provided acceptable working conditions. This measure resulted in a decrease in the number of Filipino women of 15 to 29 years who entered Japan in 1989. However, the numbers entering Japan increased considerably between 1990 and 1991 and although the figure for 1992 was lower than that of the previous year, it remained far higher than the numbers of women who had entered Japan during the previous decades.

Thailand

Whereas the Philippines has a long tradition of sending its workers to foreign countries, Thailand has a relatively short history. Thai labourers began to go to the Middle East to work in the construction sector in the early 1970s, and there was a boom in out-migration during the late 1970s (Sasaki, 1991; Yanaihara and Yamagata, 1992). These workers had originally been employed building US bases in Thailand during the Vietnam War. Before 1982, the Thai government did not have a clear policy on overseas migration. The Fifth National Economic and Social Development Plan (1982–86) included four guidelines: first, the promotion of overseas employment and the establishment of a labour office in recipient countries; second, the establishment of labour protection rules and controls over out-migration; third, skill training for workers; and fourth, the promotion of foreign currency remittances through the branches of Thai banks.

The Sixth Development Plan revealed ten new policies: the promotion of good relations with recipient countries, effective administration of overseas labour, the extension of out-migration to areas other than the Middle East, skills development for workers; skill examination and certification for workers, removal of obstacles to working abroad, reduction in the cost of out-migration, protection of workers and the punishment of illegal intermediaries, provision of information about overseas labour and intermediaries, and reception measures for workers returning to Thailand. Because Thailand started to send workers abroad relatively late, the government's measures were introduced only in recent years. Although the Thai government seems to be optimistic about its migrant workers, information about adverse working conditions in foreign countries has become available to the public, notably the case of the Thai hostesses who were arrested for murdering their boss, in a drinking bar in Japan, in order to gain their freedom.

THE DOUBLE STANDARD

Many Asian women enter Japan to work as prostitutes for economic reasons, in the context of their countries' policies for sending workers abroad. However, they would not come to Japan if there were no 'pull factors'. The demand for prostitution can be examined from both economic and social viewpoints. From an economic perspective, for example, middlemen earn considerable profits by sending South-East Asian women to work as prostitutes in Japan and Japanese men pay Asian women less than Japanese prostitutes.

It is impossible to examine this issue adequately without touching on social and cultural features of Japan. Why do men buy women? Are there any specific reasons? It is difficult to answer these questions since the explanations are complex. However, it is clear than many men buy women because they think it is normal for men to do so; at least, many men do not feel guilty about doing so. This is argued to be caused by the double standard. This section will review, historically, the creation of the double standard in Japan, focusing on prostitutes and the past and present status of Japanese women.

The Muromachi and Edo Periods

One of the first official acknowledgements of prostitution in Japan occurred during the Muromachi Period of the fifteenth and sixteenth centuries, when the Shogun government started to tax prostitution houses in Kyoto to ease its troubled financial situation. In 1590, a prostitution area was established in Kyoto by the ruler, Toyotomi, who also permitted prostitution in part of Osaka, in order to provide his followers with 'recreation and comfort'.

Japanese conservative society is said to have been established during the Edo Period (1603–1868). During this time, women's position in the family became highly vulnerable, as they lost the right to keep their own property and money. There was great pressure to maintain *ie*, the Japanese family system, and women were expected to give birth to a boy, who would become the head of a family. Men were allowed to have several wives under the pretext that families must be sustained and women were expected to be loyal to their husband so as to maintain the family blood line. Farmers' wives were subject to particular pressure as farmers were a key source of tax revenue for the Edo government, so that farmers' wives were expected to labour on the land as well as to give birth to a boy.

During the Edo Period, prostitution became more widespread (Kim, 1980). In 1617, prostitution houses were officially opened in Edo (Old Tokyo), as one of the strategies by which the government attempted to maintain its hold on power after a long period of warfare throughout Japan. The feudal lords were made to stay in Edo and encouraged to spend large sums of money in the prostitution houses, which made available prostitutes with a wide range of regional cultures. Over time, as the warrier class became less wealthy relative to the growing merchant class, the customers of the prostitution houses changed and private prostitution houses spread throughout Japan.

The Meiji Period

The Meiji government which succeeded the Edo regime introduced, in 1898, a new civil law which gave more power to the head of the household, normally a man. The law was reinforced by the education system, which taught girl students that their role was to become good housewives (Nagahara, 1982). Women were expected to obey the head of the household, married women were to change their name to that of their husband and were not allowed to engage in economic activities without their husband's permission and a husband was allowed to divorce his wife if she had extra-marital affairs while a wife could only do so if the husband's lover was married to another man who took legal action against the husband (Fukuchi, 1987). In spite of the fact that the law only permitted monogamy, children born out of wedlock were allowed to inherit the house of their father, so that the keeping of mistresses by husbands was informally accepted. Thus, the double standard, which allows men to have sexual relations outside marriage but does not permit women to do so, developed during the Edo and Meiji eras.

Divided women

The double standard also divided women into two types: women who are expected to be loyal to their husands and to be good mothers, and other women. It is not only men who accept the double standard; many women do too. Women's acceptance of the double standard has been discussed by a number of authors. For example, Usuki cites two women; one, a university student, commented 'A man who cannot have an amour is not attractive. I do not care if my boyfriend buys a girl abroad' and a wife said 'As my husband works very hard to build a new house for us and he is good to us, I allow him to have affairs' (Usuki, 1983: 96).

A conversation between two wives living in Tokyo is referred to in Kishimoto's paper:

A: My husband went on a sex tour with members of . . . cooperatives yesterday. He said that it was for socialization with other members, but I cannot stand it!

B: Well, my husband has been three times already . . . I had an argument with him in the beginning but I have already given up trying to persuade him. Men are always like that. I tolerate it so long as he doesn't get venereal diseases.

(Kishimoto, 1984: 6)

A further example of housewives who do not consider their husbands' buying prostitutes as having affairs is that of a 38-year-old wife who wrote about her husband's behaviour:

the writer noted that Nokyo (Agricultural Cooperative) has been sending what she is convinced are sex-buying group tours to Taiwan for ten years. Although she requested her husband not to join this year's tour, as a staff member of Nokyo, he felt obliged to participate. If he did not attend, he said, he would be ostracized and made to feel ashamed for giving in to his wife's demand.

(English Discussion Society, 1992: 35)

Japanese women, therefore, accept the double standard, some willingly and others unwillingly. Some were led to believe that having extra-marital affairs is natural for men and that wise women do not complain about it. Even if women doubt this norm, it is sometimes difficult for them to persuade their husbands to refrain from such behaviour.

Japanese society is changing and women of the younger generation are becoming more powerful. Some think that women, like men, should be allowed to have extra-marital affairs. It is difficult to deny that the wives mentioned above are victims of the double standard in the sense that they are expected to tolerate their husband's behaviour. However, they may also be victimizing other women by allowing men to buy other women's sexualities. Women are divided by the double standard, which allows only men to have affairs outside marriage and which classifies women into good wives and other women. Many women who are in the category of good wives find it easy to accept the norm that women who sell their bodies are a different type of woman, in a category of 'whores', racial difference making this division visible with ease.

DIFFERENCES AMONG WOMEN FROM SOUTH-EAST ASIA

Entering the 1980s, we have seen a gradual shift of prostitution away from tourist destination countries to tourists' countries of origin. As the number of sex tours has decreased, so the number of women coming to Japan from Korea, Taiwan, the Philippines and Thailand has increased. These women enter Japan with the hope of getting a better job, but in many cases they end up engaging in prostitution, often abused and exploited. However, what we should recognize is that the women from the four different countries do not have the same working conditions, nor do they engage in the same kind of jobs. It seems that their situations in Japan differ according to their nationalities.

Korean and Taiwanese women find themselves in similar situations in Japan. The number of Korean and Taiwanese women who come to Japan every year is high, as was clear from Table 7.4 on pp. 189–90. In particular, the total number of Taiwanese women entering Japan every year is between 6 per cent and 25 per cent greater than the number of Taiwanese male entrants. However, not much evidence can be found to conclude that most Korean and Taiwanese women are working as prostitutes in Japan. The statistical material 'Illegal Activities and Overstay cum Illegal Activities' published by the Japan Immigration Association indicates that some Korean and Taiwanese women work as prostitutes. For example, in 1987, 43 Korean and 196 Chinese women (including women from Taiwan, Hong Kong and mainland China) were apprehended and deported under the charge of illegally working as bar hostesses. It is often the case that bar hostesses are expected to serve as prostitutes. These numbers are rather small compared with the 5,103 Filipino and 702 Thai women apprehended during the same year under the same charge. In addition, the number of Korean and Taiwanese women going to refuges for protection is much less than that of Filipino and Thai women. A report issued by the Asian Women's Shelter HELP (House in Emergency of Love and Peace founded in 1986) informed us that they aided four Korean and five Taiwanese women from 1986 to 1993, whilst they provided support for 312 Filipino and 1103 Thai women during the same period (HELP, 1994). Although Korea and Taiwan have been two of the destination countries for Japanese sex tourism, it can be concluded that Korean and Taiwanese women do not make up the main work force of prostitutes in Japan and if any of them are engaged in prostitution, they have relatively secure working conditions.

What are the reasons for the differences between Korean and Taiwanese women on the one hand, and Filipino and Thai women on the other? They occur primarily because Korean and Taiwanese women started to come to Japan before Filipino and Thai women. Japan has had a longer relationship with both Korea and Taiwan, especially through occupying these countries before World War II and many Koreans and Taiwanese have already lived in Japan, so that women from these two countries have had easy access to Japan through their relatives or acquaintances. This entry time gap has allowed some Korean and Taiwanese women to establish some kind of status in Japanese society such as becoming a bar owner rather than a hostess or taking up permanent residence through marriage. Moreover, considering the rapidly developing economies of both Korea and Taiwan, it is reasonable to assume that not many Korean and Taiwanese women are desperate for money and willing to come to Japan as prostitutes or for a job with poor working conditions. In terms of visa status, more Koreans and Taiwanese now come to Japan on student visas than Filipinos and Thais, as indicated in Table 7.9. Nowadays, we see many young Koreans and Taiwanese studying in language schools, vocational schools and universities in Japan. Their student visas allow them to work up to four hours a day and their minimum hourly wage is guaranteed by Japanese labour law. It seems that Koreans and Taiwanese come to Japan for diverse purposes, including employment, study, vocational training and visiting relatives.

Table 7.9 The number of foreign nationals entering Japan, by nationality and visa status

Year	Taiwan Short stay	Entertainer	Student	Korea Short stay	Entertainer	Student	Philippines Short stay	Entertainer	Student	Thailand Short stay	Entertainer	Student
1987	312164	2519	10172	147958	836	8358	37311	36080	417	27430	197	844
1988	338000	2351	12296	256757	999	10886	25463	41423	546	32701	173	950
1989	443418	1970	14010	503175	1643	14586	28610	32719	695	38605	205	1049
1990	550703	2129	18595	653431	2416	31805	35701	42867	2345	57320	400	1810
1991	623168	2130	18788	769199	2837	38199	31858	57038	1587	90513	419	1945
1992	681635	1716	18644	763555	2785	42423	29404	51252	1299	81439	593	2169

Source: Annual Report of Statistics on Legal Migrants, 1988–1993, Ministry of Justice.
Note: 'Short stay' mostly denotes holidaymakers, but also includes people visiting relatives, doing business and so on for a short period.
'Student' denotes people going to high schools, vocational schools and universities.

Filipino and Thai women, who have made up the main force of prostitutes working in Japan since the 1980s, are in a different situation from Korean and Taiwanese women, and many of them have suffered severe ordeals. However, although both Filipino and Thai women have been exploited as prostitutes, the degree to which they have been abused differs. It seems that Thai women have a weaker and less secure position in Japan than Filipino women. What are the reasons for this difference? The following comparative chart of the recruitment process between Filipino and Thai women sheds some light on this issue.

The first point to consider is that Thai women go through many levels of brokers in their recruitment process and *Yakuza* gangsters are deeply involved in recruiting women to come to Japan and placing them in the entertainment industry. The *Yakuza* is a Japa-

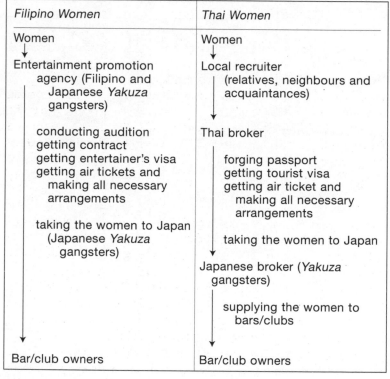

Filipino Women	Thai Women
Women ↓	Women ↓
Entertainment promotion agency (Filipino and Japanese *Yakuza* gangsters)	Local recruiter (relatives, neighbours and acquaintances) ↓
conducting audition getting contract getting entertainer's visa getting air tickets and making all necessary arrangements taking the women to Japan (Japanese *Yakuza* gangsters)	Thai broker forging passport getting tourist visa getting air ticket and making all necessary arrangements taking the women to Japan ↓ Japanese broker (*Yakuza* gangsters) supplying the women to bars/clubs ↓
Bar/club owners	Bar/club owners

Figure 7.1 Process by which Filipino and Thai women become prostitutes in Japan

nese underworld criminal syndicate which either overtly or covertly controls the management of bars and clubs in most of the entertainment districts of Japan. In the case of Filipino women, they must sign a contract through entertainment promotion agencies in the Philippines in order to apply for a visa. At first, the agencies were run by local Filipino people but soon *Yakuza* gangsters started to join in the process of choosing women at audition times. Then, the gangsters took the women to Japan and earned commission by placing them in bars and clubs in the entertainment districts of big cities or spa resorts in the countryside. They sometimes let the women work in bars which they or their common-law wives run. Apart from their legitimate jobs as show dancers or singers, the Filipino women are often forced by the bar or club owners to become involved in prostitution. If a woman spends the night with a client, she can earn 100,000 yen whilst the bar owner receives 200,000 yen from the client (Ohshima and Francis, 1989: 29).

Soon, the *Yakuza* gangsters found another target for exploitation. They discovered that they could easily make a larger amount of profit from Thai women. Although we see many Filipino dancers in the entertainment districts of Japan, they are not so visible as prostitutes nowadays. Instead, we see many Thai women working as prostitutes in bars, clubs and on the streets. Judging from the statistics issued by the refuge centre, HELP, the shift happened sometime around 1988. Is it a coincidence that the Thai government launched a campaign called 'Visit Thailand Year' in order to promote tourism in its country that year? The statistics published by HELP indicate that the majority of women coming to the refuge for protection were Filipino women up until 1987, but from the next year their numbers decreased considerably. Conversely, the number of Thai women seeking protection rose from nine in 1987 to 144 in 1988 and the number has continued to increase during the 1990s. Statistics issued by a refuge called Women's House *Sala* show a similar tendency; two Filipino women and 54 Thai women had used the refuge out of the total 56 women during the period from September 1992 to April 1993. These women are, of course, a tiny minority of the women who work as prostitutes in Japan.

It is reported that two different underworld criminal syndicates are involved in sending Thai women to Japan, Chinese syndicates on the side of Thailand and *Yakuza* syndicates on the Japanese side (Asian Women's Association, 1992; Tezuka, 1992; Yamatani,

1992). The syndicates in Thailand have already established the means of recruiting young women from poor farming areas and sending them overseas. They use local people as recruitment agents to collect women, and then members of the syndicates forge passports, make all the necessary arrangements, take the women to Japan and hand them over to Japanese brokers, mostly *Yakuza* gangsters, who pay between 1.5 and 1.8 million yen per woman as commission to a Thai broker. The Japanese brokers place the women in bars and clubs all over Japan and charge 3 to 3.5 million yen as commission for the women. The bar/club owners add some extra money to the commission and tell the woman that they have a 'debt' of 3.5 to 4 million yen to repay. It is the women who have to bear the entire cost. The Thai women are burdened with an enormous debt which they work to repay, although there are no legal grounds on which they have to repay it. The system of recruiting Thai women for Japanese bars and clubs can be identified as human trafficking and the women are confined and exploited within the system. It is obvious that the recruiters, brokers and bar owners are making huge profits by sending Thai women to Japan.

The second point to consider is the visa status of the women. The Philippines government's policy of encouraging people to get jobs overseas as a means of expanding employment opportunities and gaining foreign currency to accelerate the growth of the economy was discussed above. Filipino women are not the exception under this policy. When they try to look for jobs in Japan, they face a big obstacle: closed labour markets for overseas workers in Japan. Japan follows the policy of accepting only specialists from overseas, not simple manual labourers such as factory or construction site workers, waiters or waitresses and shop clerks. The entertainer's visa seems to be the only legitimate working visa which most young Filipino women can obtain without much trouble, as indicated in Table 7.9. The entertainer's visa at least guarantees their security to some extent. Obtaining an entertainer's visa requires a proper contract which stipulates wage and accommodation conditions, the name of the responsible agent and so on. It also allows the holder to stay in Japan legally for up to 180 days. As a contracted worker, she is entitled to appeal for legal protection or bring an action against her employer in the case of contractual violation. However, in practice, such prosecutions are not always easy to undertake because of the difficulty in obtaining enough evidence. For example, women who run away from their employers usually do not carry their contract with them, so that it is hard for them to prove the name of their employers or the place where they worked. On the other hand, the majority of Thai women come to Japan on short stay visas (see Table 7.9). A short stay visa is the easiest type to obtain for entry from overseas but does not allow the holder to work or stay in Japan for more than 90 days. Hence, those women entering Japan on tourist visas have no means of looking for a job openly by them- selves and if they do something for money, they fall into the category of illegal workers so that they cannot rely on any legal protection and rather try to hide themselves from the public sphere due to the fear of deportation. Taking advantage of the Thai women's insecure status in Japan, *Yakuza* gangsters and bar owners make use of the women, who usually work in particularly adverse conditions, to gain an easy profit.

The third point to consider is the degree of their self-help. Both Filipino and Thai women do not usually speak Japanese, so they do not easily understand what is happening around them. How- ever, most Filipino women speak English, in which they can communicate with the local Japanese when necessary. Thai women often only speak their own language so they tend to be more isolated and have less access to information. Moreover, compared with Filipino women, Thai women are more restricted in their daily behaviour. For example, they are not allowed to go anywhere by themselves, even to a nearby shop. They are always under close watch of their employers. Therefore, even in times of emergency, it is difficult for them to contact someone for help. Filipino women have a further advantage over Thai women. Because they are usually Catholics, they tend to go to church regularly, which enables them to make friends, exchange informa- tion and set up support groups if they wish, or to obtain help from church officials and local churchgoers.

WOMEN'S EXPERIENCES: THE CASE OF THAI WOMEN

Women engaging in prostitution have a wide range of different experiences. Some are successful in saving up large amounts of money to take back home and others run away from their owners and come to a refuge for protection or end up in terrible hardship. What is common among them is that they have little power to negotiate their working conditions with their brokers or bar/club owners. The following is a typical example of a Thai woman's experience of coming to Japan and engaging in sex work. The story is based on one of the interviews I conducted in 1993 with the help of an interpreter. The Thai woman, called 'M', was 26 years old and started working in a bar in Tokyo in December 1991. She wanted to remain anonymous because she was afraid of the consequences that might occur because of the interview.

M decided to come to Japan after being invited by a woman living next door. She went from a small village near Chiang Mai in the north of Thailand to Bangkok and worked as a shop clerk after graduating from a vocational school. At the time when M heard about the job opportunity in Japan, she was very depressed after losing her boyfriend and wanted to go somewhere far away. Although her parents disagreed with her decision and she was told she would have a debt of 3.6 million yen to pay off in Japan, she did not change her mind. She was worried at first that 3.6 million yen was a lot of money, but was told that it would only take 3 months to pay back. Someone arranged to get hold of a passport for her, which was a forgery. She came to Japan on a tourist visa escorted by a Thai man who took her from Bangkok to a bar in Tokyo. M was told by the *Mama-san* who ran the bar to start working from the next day, also that she was indeed 3.8 million yen in debt. The *Mama-san* was Taiwanese.

When she first started working, there were 20 other women working in the bar as hostesses and at the same time as prostitutes but in 1994 eleven women (nine from Thailand, one from Hong Kong and one from Taiwan) were working there. All the women working in the bar had to live above the bar, until they became free by paying off their debt. It took five months for her to repay the debt including an extra 20 thousand yen for moving to a new apartment. Her clients were mostly in their 40s and she felt some of them treated her very badly. After she became free, she continued to work for the bar on an unpaid basis but was allowed to receive the full charge for her sexual service and kept working in the same bar to save money for her parents and herself. Her parents, sister and her sister's husband built a new house with the money she sent them and are now living there together. She said that she does not want to go back to Thailand because Tokyo is more exciting and there are a lot more things to do and see than in Bangkok. Some of her clients took her for day excursions or trips of a few days, and the most impressive trip for her was going to Sapporo for the Snow

Festival. She now has a Japanese boyfriend, a sugar daddy, who gives her some money so that she has not engaged in prostitution for the last three months.

Until they finish paying off their debt, Thai women receive no money from the work they do. Only a tip from their clients makes up the income at their disposal. They are provided with food and a place to live by the bar owners but in many cases the owners do so to prevent the women from going out freely. Sometimes bar owners calculate the daily expenses of a woman and add them to her debt. Another Thai woman, called 'S', said that she was told to pay 50 thousand yen as a housing fee every month on top of her debt after she had worked for five months. If a woman takes a day off, she is usually fined 10 thousand yen, which is added to her debt. It is said that it costs 15–20 thousand yen for a few hours or 25–30 thousand yen to stay overnight with a prostitute on average. M worked off the debt in five months, which means she had a client nearly every day during that period. S has not yet paid off the debt of 3.9 million yen, even though she has worked for about ten months.

In contrast to Filipino women who sometimes take tourists as clients because they work as show dancers at hotels in resorts, Thai women usually work for local bars and therefore most of their clients are local men living in the vicinity, aged 'mainly from 30 to 50 years old and married', according to a bar owner whom I interviewed. There are cities and towns in Japan which have entertainment districts where many Thai women work. Big factory compounds, large construction sites or an army post of the self-defence force are often located there. Hence, these cities and towns have many unmarried men or married men separated from their families, gathered together for work, and prostitutes accommodate their demands. In cities like Tokyo, entertainment districts are scattered in several different areas and it is rare to see Thai women working in bars and clubs in such a top area as 'Ginza' where high class company executives entertain their important business customers and Japanese bar hostesses predominate. Thai women said that some clients were nice and gave them a lot of money and others were cruel. For example, S spent a night with a client who terrified her by putting a 'long knife' near the bed and saying that he was always ready to use it if she did not obey him.

When women have finished working off their debt and become independent, they rarely go back home straight away. Instead, they try their best to earn and save money for themselves or their families through working for the same bars independently, moving to other bars with better conditions or becoming streetwalkers. As street-walkers, they can work as freelance prostitutes but inevitably take the risk of being easy targets for police discipline and *Yakuza* gangsters' demands to act as pimps. On the whole, the future of women without debts is to go back home with some money saved, to stay in Japan continuing to work as a prostitute, to become the mistress of, or get married to, a Japanese man, or to become agents or brokers who recruit women to Japan.

WOMEN'S RESPONSES

Prostitution is often criticized at both personal and institutional levels as an immoral and anti-social activity. The South-East Asian countries from which the women come often have Buddhist, Catho-lic or Confucian faiths that condemn prostitution as a shameful form of behaviour. The women are, therefore, constantly under psycho-logical pressure. An activist of a support group said that about one-third of the women coming to Japan knew, beforehand, that they would be working as prostitutes in Japan. The rest of the women had no choice but to accept the work even though they found out after arriving in Japan that they had been deceived. S said 'One of my acquaintances invited me to work in Japan as a waitress. When I was told to work as a prostitute, I didn't know what to do and where to go, so I accepted the work. I had already come to Japan, so what could I do?' Most of the women accept prostitution as a means of survival; survival for themselves and their families back home. Even though they cannot escape feelings of shame, they have pride in the fact that they support themselves and contribute to the sustenance of their families.

On the other hand, there are many women whose lives have been devastated by their experience. Some have risked their lives by running away from their bar owners and have gone to a refuge for protection or to their embassy for help. It is reported that the Thai Embassy in Tokyo dealt with about 3,000 Thai women who sought help in 1991 and with 3,000–3,500 every month in 1992 (Matsui, 1993b). The non-governmental refuge HELP provided a refuge for 1,170 Thai and Filipino women from 1987 to 1992, *Sala* helped 56 women during nine months in 1993, and *Mizura* aided 67 Thai women between 1992 and 1993. Criminal offences in which Thai women are either the offender or victim are increasing, too. Between January and September, 1992, there were 57 criminal offences involving Thai women and 397 Thai women were arrested or placed under police protection (*Yomiuri* newspaper, 2 October 1992). Amongst the offences, three murder cases stand out and highlight the plight of South-East Asian women working in Japan.

The first case is that of three women on trial for killing their Thai female boss in Shimodate, Ibaragi Prefecture. The second is that of six women, including a 15-year-old girl, accused of killing their bar owner, a Taiwanese woman, in Shinkoiwa, Tokyo. The third is that of five women on trial for killing their bar owner, a Singapore woman, in Mobara, Chiba Prefecture. According to the women's testimony and letters to their support groups, they committed the killings because they wanted to escape from the bars. They had believed they were going to work in factories or restaurants until they came to Japan but in reality they were forced to engage in prostitution. On their arrival, they were told to pay back 3.8 million yen and their passports were taken away. Some were told that if they ran away or did not do what they were told, their parents would be killed. Others were stripped of their clothes, photographed and told that the photographs would be sent to Thai newspapers if they misbehaved. They were fined for speaking in their own language, smoking, not smiling and not giving adequate service to customers in the bars. The women in the Mobara case were told to do everything that their clients wanted. For example, an overnight engagement of sexual services means having sexual intercourse several times and having to massage the clients until morning, and the women are not allowed to sleep during the night (Hand-in-Hand Chiba, 1994: 22). They were like prisoners, having no freedom to go out by themselves. One of the women wrote a letter from a Detention Centre saying:

There was no factory where I could work in Japan, but only pubs and bars. There were only men who thought about nothing more than getting drunk and having sex with strangers. For me every day was suffering. I had to sleep with men whom I did not know at all. If I did not obey the orders of the manager of the bar I was beaten. For the Japanese masters, women from Thailand are considered to be lower than animals.

(Hand-in-Hand Chiba, 1993: 31)

CONCLUSION

Prostitution tourism is a product which has evolved from the inter-play between political, social, cultural and economic factors. Since the 1960s, tourism has been promoted under government leadership as an important part of the development of the nations in the South-East Asian region. This policy of promoting tourism induced a massive growth of prostitution, with large numbers of men coming from industrialized countries across the world. Because of the vicinity and economic power of Japan, together with their cultural expectations that women be submissive, Japanese men were among the most dominant tourists in search of sexual pleasure in those countries.

Campaigns against prostitution tourism were stimulated by the criticisms voiced by the Christian Women's Federation of Korea in 1973 and gained further momentum when the National Christian Council (NCC), its branch organization the Japan Women's Christian Temperance Union (JWCTU) and other women's groups joined together in publishing research papers, visiting travel companies, making slides to reveal the activities of Japanese sex tour groups and protesting to the Ministry of Transportation. They also developed a campaign to coordinate with women's groups in the Philippines and Thailand and, as a result, when Prime Minister Suzuki visited ASEAN countries in 1981, he met large demonstrations in each country. However, as travel companies started refraining from organizing sex tour groups after facing considerable protest movements in the 1970s, prostitution spread from the tourist destination countries to tourist origin countries, including Japan, and has spread widely over the country. Why was this shift possible? What are the reasons and factors underpinning the phenomenon and what are some of the possible ways of improving the women's situations?

First of all, the focus should be on the great material differences in wealth between the nations. Japan is extremely wealthy compared with the other four countries in terms of income per capita. The strong economic power of Japan is also reflected in the exchange rate of Japanese currency. Since 1985, the exchange rate of the Japanese yen against other currencies has appreciated dramatically, providing workers paid in yen with a huge increase in their purchasing power. As a result, Japan has attracted migrant workers from many developing countries in South-East Asia, the Middle East and South America. The flow of women from South-East

Asian countries is, thus, not an isolated phenomenon in the context of the world economy. On the other hand, taking advantage of their affluent economic status, Japanese go to luxurious resorts for rest and leisure and sometimes associate with prostitutes. In the case of prostitution involving South-East Asian women, it is clear that international disparities in power and wealth determine who is doing the buying and who is selling.

Second, we should consider the interrelationships between material interests and political power. In the cases of both Filipino and Thai women who come to Japan, most work for their own sustenance and that of their families and wish to obtain a better standard of living. Thus, the number of women who want to work in Japan will not decrease so long as poverty is not irradicated in their home countries. For example, expensive houses stand in the middle of some poor farming villages in Thailand and the owners of these houses have daughters working in Japan. It is possible for women to earn a large amount of money in a relatively short period through prostitution in Japan. In fact, they can earn much more in Japan than they would earn by doing the same job in their home countries. However, it is the intermediaries who benefit most by using the women and have real power to control the situation. In the case of Thai women, in particular, recruiters, brokers, agents and bar owners make extremely high amounts of commission through the process of transporting women. In the end, women are told to pay off about 3.5–4 million yen, which is equivalent to £20,000–£22,800. Until they work off the debt, they are resigned to their powerless position and receive no wages for the job they do.

In addition, clients benefit from South-East Asian women prostitutes because the majority seem to charge less for their sexual services than Japanese women. The district and the types of establishment in which they work are different. For example, we can see only Japanese women working in bars and clubs in Tokyo's most expensive neighbourhood, demonstrating both racist and class overtones in the demand for prostitution. The women from South-East Asian countries can be found in less expensive areas of Tokyo and local cities which are full of cheaper drinking places. This means that Japanese men, as clients, spend less for their sexual pleasure.

Third, we should address socio-cultural factors in Japanese society, where many women have been accepted as prostitutes. Historically, prostitution has been used to satisfy and control male sexuality. Japanese society has been tolerant towards, or sometimes praised, men's promiscuity in so far as they keep households secure. On the other hand, women are divided into two categories: virtuous daughters and wives, and 'whores'. Women in the former category are required to give their absolute loyalty to their fathers and husbands after marriage. Women in the latter category are regarded as outcasts of society, segregated into special quarters for the sake of protecting public morality and accommodating men's sexual needs. This tradition allowed the establishment of a series of prostitution systems in the past such as the state-regulated prostitution system inherited from the late sixteenth century and abolished as late as 1946 by the disuse of the Regulation of the Control of Shougi (a kind of Geisha), the comfort women drafted into sexual slavery by the Imperial Army during World War II, and the Recreation and Amusement Association (RAA) established to accommodate the sexual needs of the soldiers in the Occupation Army. In the same way, South-East Asian women are accepted into Japanese society as a means of controlling and satisfying male sexuality, and yet they are shunned by mainstream society and treated as outcasts.

Traditions persist. To some extent, both Japanese men and women cannot be free from traditional values. Under the remaining influence of the absolute power traditionally given to the head of the family, there are still many Japanese men who hold traditional ideas about women's submissiveness and obedience towards them and South-East Asian women are often told to satisfy those demands. The women accept the demands without being able to protest because of their powerless situation. The ambivalent attitude taken by Japanese wives also reveals the fact that they are still confined by tradition in wondering on what basis they can complain about their husbands' conduct in so far as their husbands fulfil their roles in the family as heads of households and breadwinners. Tradition tells us to be tolerant of men's promiscuity. Many Japanese wives would conclude that buying prostitutes is just temporary, after all, because prostitutes belong to a different group of women and it is pointless to risk the family's security and stability by complaining too much about their husband's unfaithful behaviour. However, this attitude emphasizes the material aspect of the couple's relationship and diminishes the spiritual aspect. Mutual trust and respect are also important components in maintaining the couple's relationship but tend to be forgotten. Such a materialistic ideology and double standard allows people to be blind to the fact that prostitutes have their own families at home and engage in sex work on behalf of their families.

The legal approach towards prostitution in Japan prescribed in the current Prostitution Prevention Law should be re-examined. The Law was enacted in 1956 and consists of two components. One is concerned with penalization of acts. The name of the Law states 'prevention' and not 'prohibition' and the objective of the Law is not to penalize the act of prostitution itself but to impose a penalty on any acts which encourage and promote prostitution, such as soliciting in public and procuring women for prostitution. The second component is concerned with establishing facilities for counselling and the rehabilitation of prostitutes. However, the Law has three main defects in the administration of justice for women working as prostitutes.

First, it lacks effective measures for penalizing procurers operating today, particularly regarding procurement of women from South-East Asia. Under the Law, it is possible to prosecute bar owners in charge of procurement for prostitution but, in practice, such prosecution is hard to undertake because the women do not wish to get involved in law suits due to their illegal status in Japan. Besides, even if a woman running away from her bar owner wishes to make a prosecution with the help of a lawyer, the attempt is usually in vain because she cannot prove where she worked and the name of the bar owner for whom she worked. The primary problem in prostitution within Japan itself is the serious degree of exploitation by bar owners as procurers of women. It is urgent that effective measures are taken to punish procurers.

Second, making soliciting an offence works against women. It is always prostitutes who are arrested and charged and men's kerb-crawling or looking for a prostitute goes unquestioned. Nowadays, the main target of police operations are Thai women who become free from their procurers and work on the streets for themselves. In order to end this one-sided administration of the Law, there are two points to be considered: one is the question of establishing some measures to impose a penalty on men's kerb-crawling and the other is to rethink the necessity of Article 5 of the Law, which states that soliciting should be penalized.

Third, although the counselling and rehabilitation scheme is an important component of the Law and could provide good opportunities for indicating alternative options to prostitutes, women from South-East Asia have no chance of benefiting from the scheme unless they hold a legally valid visa, otherwise they will be sent to the Bureau of Immigration Control for deportation. Language is also a big barrier to women's ability to make use of the opportunities. Furthermore, facilities for the scheme are in danger of being run down because of the government's limited financial support. We should pressurize the government to provide more finance to revitalize such schemes and, at the same time, it is important to ensure that the rehabilitation programmes truly respond to women's needs today.

In addition to the above three defects, it is necessary to re-examine the effect of the conventional approach towards prostitution. The anti-prostitution movement in Japan was launched more than a hundred years ago under the leadership of Christian organizations such as the JWCTU, founded in 1886, and the Salvation Army, founded in 1895. The movement has made a significant contribution towards abolishing state-regulated prostitution, providing relief and rehabilitation facilities for prostitutes and formulating government policies on prostitution. Their activities have been conducted with the aim of the total abolition of prostitution, presuming that prostitution is offensive and exploitative towards women. It is clear that they have condemned not the individual prostitutes, but the practice of prostitution as an institution. However, their stance entails a rather negative attitude towards prostitutes, regarding them as passive victims who should be guided and saved. How far is this approach consistent with the reality of South-East Asian women working as prostitutes in Japan? Prostitution enables the women to obtain a large amount of money which is necessary for their livelihood and that of their families and, despite all the exploitative working conditions, many women still choose to work as prostitutes. Therefore, it is important to investigate the possibility of a form of prostitution permitted by society, in which the prostitutes' human rights are not violated.

The issues of prostitution tourism cannot be solved by a domestic solution alone, but require internationally coordinated action. As we have seen, the expansion of tourism has brought about the proliferation of prostitution in South-East Asia. Such a social change in the region seems to be interlocked with the increasing entry of South-East Asian women into Japan and their resulting powerless situation. The national development strategies currently taken in the region need to be reconsidered not only in the light of the enrichment of the nations but also in the light of reducing the economic disparity within the nations. A microeconomic perspective is more relevant in alleviating the hardship that South-East Asian women are facing than a macroeconomic approach. It is important that overseas development aid from Japan to the developing countries in the region should be coordinated towards empowering individuals.

REFERENCES

Asian Women's Association (ed.) (1992) *Asian Women's Liberation. Thai josei wa naze Nihon ni?* (Why do Thai women come to Japan?) *Asian Women's Liberation*, no. 21, November, Tokyo.

Awanohara, S. (1975) 'Protesting the sexual imperialists', *Far Eastern Economic Review*, vol. 87, no. 11, 14 March: 5–6.

Cohen, E. (1982) 'Thai girls and farang men. The edge of ambiguity', *Annals of Tourism Research* 9: 403–28.

English Discussion Society (ed.) (1992) *Japanese Women Now*, Kyoto: Women's Bookstore Shoukadoh.

Findley, S. and Williams, L. (1991) *Women Who Go and Women Who Stay: Reflections of Family Migration Processes in a Changing World*, Working Paper 176, Geneva: International Labour Organisation.

Fukuchi, S. (1987) *Kindai Nihon Joseishi* (Modern History of Japanese Women), Tokyo: Sekkasha.

Hall, C.M. (1992) 'Sex tourism in South-east Asia', in D. Harrison (ed.) *Tourism and the Less Developed Countries*, London: Belhaven.

Hand-in-Hand Chiba (ed.) (1993) *Report Mobara Jiken* (The Report on the Mobara Case), Chiba: Hand-in-Hand Chiba.

Hand in Hand Chiba (ed.) (1994) *Zoku Report Mobara Jiken* (The Second Report on the Mobara Case), Chiba: Hand-in-Hand Chiba.

Handley, P. (1989) 'The lust frontier', *Far Eastern Economic Review*, vol. 146, no. 44, 2 November: 44–5.

HELP (1994) *Network News*, Asian Women's Shelter HELP, no. 27, 10 May: 4.

Heyzer, N. (1986) *Working Women in South-East Asia Development, Subordination and Emancipation*, Milton Keynes: Open University Press.

Hiebert, M. and Ladd, G. (1993) 'Flower-sellers' bloom', *Far Eastern Economic Review*, vol. 156, no. 27, 8 July: 36.

ISIS (Inter Cultural Studies Information Service) (1979) 'Tourism and Prostitution', Special Issue of *ISIS International Bulletin*, 13.

Japan Travel Bureau (1991) *Ryokou Nenpo* (Annual Report on Travelling), Japan: Japan Travel Bureau.

Kelly, N. (1991) 'Counting the cost', *Far Eastern Economic Review*, vol. 153, no. 29, 18 July: 44.

Kim, Il Meng (1980) *Nihon Josei Aishi* (Sad History of Japanese Women), Tokyo: Tokuma Shoten.

Kishimoto, K. (1984) 'Watashi-tachi wa Ajia no minshu no rinjin to naranakereba naranai' (We should be good neighbours to Asian people), *Fujin Shimpo*, no. 7, Tokyo.

Lee, W. (1991) 'Prostitution and tourism in South-East Asia', in N. Redclift and M.T. Sinclair (eds) *Working Women, International Perspectives on Labour and Gender Ideology*, London and New York: Routledge, (Japanese translation *Gender and Women's Labour*, Tokyo: Tuge Shobe, 1994).

Matsui, Y. (1991) 'Asian migrant women working at sex industry in Japan victimized by international trafficking', in K. Srisang *et al.* (eds) *Caught in Modern Slavery: Tourism and Child Prostitution in Asia*, Bangkok: The Ecumenical Coalition on Third World Tourism.

Matsui, Y. (1993a) *Aija no Kanko Kaihatsu to Nihon* (Japan and the Development of Tourism in Asia), Tokyo: Shinkan sha.

Matsui, Y. (1993b) 'Nandemo Q & A: jinshin baibai 1' (Question and answer for everything: human trafficking 1), *Asahi Newspaper*, 16 March.

Mingmongkol, S. (1981) 'Official blessings for the "Brothel of Asia"', *Southeast Asia Chronicle*, no. 78: 24–25.

Ministry of Justice (1965–1993) *Annual Report of Statistics on Legal Migrants*, Tokyo: Ministry of Justice, Judicial System and Research Department, Minister's Secretariat.

Miyoshi, A. (1986) 'Firipin josei no dekasegi' (Migration of Filipino women), *Fujin Shimpo*, no. 1026: 16–20, Tokyo.

Nagahara, K. (1982) 'Ryosai kenbo shugi kyoiku ni okeru Ie to shokugyo' (The Japanese family and occupation within education to make a good wife and wise mother), in Josei-shi Sogo Kenyukai (Women's History Study Group) (ed.) *Nihon Josei-shi 4*, Tokyo: University of Tokyo Press.

Office of the National Economic and Social Development Board (1990) *National Income of Thailand*, Bangkok: NESDB.

Ogawa, M. (1985) 'Dogo onsen de Japayuki baishun tekihatsu' (Japayuki prostitutes arrested at Dogo spa), *Fujin Shimpo*, no. 1020: 26, Tokyo.

O'Grady, R. (1981) *Third World Stopover: The Tourism Debate*, Geneva: World Council of Churches.

O'Grady, R. (1992) *The Child and the Tourists*, End Child Prostitution in Asian Tourism (ECPAT): Bangkok.

O'Grady, R. (1994) *The Rape of the Innocent*, ECPAT: Bangkok in association with Pace Publishing: Auckland.

Ohshima, S. and Francis, C. (1989) *Japan through the Eyes of Women Migrant Workers*, Tokyo: Japan Women's Christian Temperance Union.

Phongpaichit, P. (1982) *From Peasant Girls to Bangkok Masseuses*, Geneva: ILO Women, Work and Development Series, no. 2.

Richter, L. (1980) 'The political uses of tourism: a Philippines case study', *The Journal of Developing Areas*, vol. 14: 237–57.

Richter, L. (1981) 'Tourism by decree', *Southeast Asia Chronicle*, no. 78: 27–32.

Sasaki, S. (1991) *Aija Kara Fuko Kaze* (Wind from Asia), Tokyo: Asahi Shimbun.

Srisang, K., Srisang, S., Rogers, J., Sexton, S., Wiebe, C., Tananone, B. and O'Grady, A. (eds) (1991) *Caught in Modern Slavery: Tourism and Child*

Prostitution in Asia, Bangkok: The Ecumenical Coalition on Third World Tourism.

Statistics Office of the Republic of the Philippines (1989) *Statistical Yearbook of the Philippines*, Manila: Statistics Office of the Republic of the Philippines.

Takazato, K. (1983) 'Nihon-no baishun kanko' (Sex tourism in Japan), in R. O'Grady (ed.) *Ajia-no-Kanko Kogai* (The Contaminating Aspects of Tourism in Asia), Tokyo: Kyobun-kan.

Takigawa, T. (ed.) (1985) *Shin-Tonan Ajia Handbook* (New Handbook of Southeast Asia), Tokyo: Kodansha.

Tezuka, C. (1992) *Tai Kara Kita Josei Tachi* (Women from Thailand), Tokyo: San'itsu Shinsho.

Tomioka, Y. (1990) *Tai-Shokan: Isan no Onna-Tachi* (Women in Isaan), Tokyo: Gendai Shokan.

Truong, T-D. (1983) 'The dynamics of sex tourism: the case of Southeast Asia', *Development and Change*, vol. 14, no. 4: 533–53.

United Nations Population Fund (1993) *The State of World Population*, New York: United Nations.

Usuki, K. (1983) *Gendai no Ianfu Tachi* (Comfort Women Now), Tokyo: Tokuma Shoten.

Utsumi, A. and Matsui, Y. (1988) *Ajia Kara Kita Rodosha-tachi* (Workers from Asia), Tokyo: Akashi Shoten.

Villariba, M.C. (1993) *Canvasses of Women in the Philippines*, International Report 7, London: CHANGE.

Wood, R.E. (1981) 'The economics of tourism', *Southeast Asia Chronicle*, No. 78: 2–9.

World Bank (1973) *World Bank Atlas*, Washington: World Bank.

World Bank (1982, 1993) *World Development Report*, Washington: World Bank.

Yamaguchi, A. (1980) 'Saishu-to kanko no soshi-wo' (Stop tours to Chejudo Island), *Fujin Shimpo* no. 960: 13, Tokyo.

Yamatani, T. (1992) *Japayuki-san: Onnatachi no Ajia* (Japayuki-san: Women's Asia), Tokyo: Kodansya.

Yanaihara, M. and Yamagata, T. (eds) (1992) *Ajia no Kokusai Rodo Ido* (Migration of Labourers within Asia), Tokyo: Ajia Keizai Kenkyujo.

Chapter 8

Gendered work in tourism
Comparative perspectives

M. Thea Sinclair

INTRODUCTION

Previous contributions to the literature on gender and tourism have described the segmented structure of work in tourism, considered some of the effects of tourism on gender roles and discussed the issue of prostitution tourism (for example, Kinnaird and Hall, 1994; Swain, 1995). The authors in this book extend the literature by focusing particularly on the theme of gender and work, complementing their descriptions of the structuring of work with analyses of the nature and effects of gendered workforce divisions. The issue of gender and work is not only of theoretical interest but of practical relevance. Gender differences are associated with inequalities between men and women, and policies and campaigns which aim to confront these inequalities incorporate assumptions about the nature of gender definitions and the reasons for their persistence or change. By examining the gendered structuring of work in tourism and its underlying rationales, the contributors to this book provide the basis for the formulation of strategies for confronting them effectively.

The methodologies which were used by the contributors who carried out studies involving interviews are related to feminist standpoint theory in so far as they take account of women's experiences using the women's own accounts, which are examined within a wider economic and social context (Smith, 1987). Standpoint theory rejects a positivist conception of knowledge but is not committed to a specific branch of feminism (Ramazanoglu, 1989). Cultural relativists have accused standpoint theory of providing a range of different and sometimes contradictory experiences from which it is impossible to select a representative account. The authors within this book avoided this critique by their acknowledgement of diversity among women and the fact that different women's experiences are shaped by their individual social and economic contexts. Hence, explicit recognition of diversity is a positive feature of the studies. The empirical research was interactive and many of the relationships made between the contributors and the women and men they interviewed are ongoing. The choice of methodology and subject matter by all the contributors was related not only to their beliefs that their personal interactions with and accounts of women's and men's work in tourism would provide much fuller and more accurate explanations of interrelationships within the sector; it was also related to their own positions as women who are actively working towards the elimination of gender inequality.

The issues which were examined in the book include the nature and effects of the gender structuring of work within household-based enterprises and large firms. The contributors also considered the ways in which norms of social sexuality can act as a constraint on women's access to jobs and social interactions with tourists or determine the type of work and social relations in which they are expected to engage. The authors identified material and ideological factors which contribute to the formation and persistence of gender definitions and associated labour force divisions or to changes in them. The types and effects of changes which have occurred in the context of tourism have been discussed and the issue of diversity and difference among women explored. The following section examines the ways in which the contributions in this book shed light on this range of issues, discussed in more detail in Chapter 1.

COMPARATIVE PERSPECTIVES ON GENDER AND WORK

Concepts of gender and social sexuality are formed, in part, by representations of women and men in advertising media. There has been some debate about the ways in which women have been represented in tourism marketing. On the one hand, a number of authors have argued that women have been objectified by the media so that male consumers perceive their holidays as including the consumption of exotic sexuality. Thus Momsen, for example, argues that 'The tourist image portrayed in the source countries is still one of scantily clad, young women in exotic surroundings appealing to the fantasies of middle-aged businessmen who are feeling threatened by the empowerment of women in the North' (1994: 117). Similar arguments have been put forward by Davidson (1985), Enloe (1989) and Lee (1991) in the context of prostitution tourism. Cohen (1995) showed how tourism publicity for the British Virgin Islands involves sexual imagery, within which women are represented as the exotic 'other', while Edensor and Kothari (1994) demonstrated the ways in which masculine images dominate interpretations of heritage in Stirling. However, Buck (1977) and Dilley (1986) found that sexualized representations did not appear to be prevalent in tour operators' brochures.

Margaret Marshment's study of representation in a wide range of UK tour operators' brochures supports the view that women are not generally portrayed as sexual objects. This is also the case for brochures produced by tour operators from other west European countries. UK tour operators provide a range of brochures which are directed towards different socio-economic classes, with alternative levels of spending power, and holiday representations tend to be based around the couple or a stereotypical nuclear family. As Marshment points out, women are assumed to be able to take their holidays on the same basis as men and the representations of women within brochures imply 'the domestication of her sexuality within the family'. Tourists are portrayed as white, able-bodied and heterosexual so that the brochures support dominant ideological norms concerning heterosexual relationships. Japanese tour operators' brochures, somewhat paradoxically, portray tourists as European rather than Japanese.

Marshment, like Urry (1990), found few examples of black tourists and it is only in brochures marketing long-haul destinations that non-whites appear, generally being portrayed in roles of serving tourists, as waiters, shopkeepers and entertainers, or in representations of such traditional working situations as fishing or agriculture. The residents of tourist destination countries are not depicted within a family or sexualized context but aestheticized representations of women are instead included, evoking sentiments of friendliness and safety. Thus, Marshment showed that it is not appropriate to assume that women are sexually commoditized within representation. Gender depictions instead associate femininity with non-sexualized pleasure, safety and security. The actual roles of women within their work contexts in tourist destinations were examined in the ensuing chapters.

The relative stability of gender divisions in the UK tourism workforce over the past decade was demonstrated by Kate Purcell. Women's employment is concentrated particularly in accommodation and catering, whereas men predominate in the transportation sector. A considerably greater proportion of women than men work on a part-time basis, women's wages are significantly lower than men's and fewer women than men are managers. Purcell paid particular attention to examining the reasons why women are recruited to specific jobs by considering the characteristics of different occupations within the economy. Contingently gendered jobs are those for which the demand for labour is gender-neutral; employers require a low wage labour force and are indifferent as to the gender of those who undertake the specified tasks. Women supply much of the low wage labour and provide additional qualities of commitment and reliability. The second occupational category is termed sex-typed occupations, for which employers demand labour with gendered attributes. Workers are required to behave according to prescribed codes of conduct and women's work sometimes involves sexualized modes of behaviour. Thus, the demand and supply characteristics of women's labour tend to be mutually reinforcing. This type of labour corresponds most closely to patriarchal capitalist relations.

Patriarchally prescribed occupations are the third category. Employers and managers demand women's labour in conjunction with that of their male partner, the condition of gendered characteristics of work being attached to the labour of each party. However, the employment contract is made with the male partner so that women's work is not subject to wage relations. Thus, women's access to and conditions of work are determined, to a great extent, by their male partners, employers and managers. Work in public houses is an interesting example of this type of production (Adkins, 1995). Purcell's empirical evidence concerning the careers of male and female students who completed hotel and catering management courses in the UK does not support the theory that women can improve their positions in accommodation and catering via increased education and training. Such 'supply-side improvements' do not generally result in higher earnings and positions for women in the occupational hierarchy of the hospitality sector.

The structure of the accommodation sector in Northern Cyprus is characterized by a significant proportion of family-based guesthouses relative to large hotels and Julie Scott examined work relations in the different types of enterprise. Patriarchal relations dominate tourism service provision in small accommodation enterprises. Turkish Cypriot women may undertake some of the cooking and cleaning, which is most closely connected to their domestic role. However, the *namus* honour–shame code, which regulates women's interactions with those other than kin, ensures that social and business contacts are carried out by men. Since much of the work which women undertake is not subject to wage relations, material forces do not play a significant role in changing women's position and the relationship between the division of labour in small tourism enterprises and the ideology of social sexuality tends to be mutually reinforcing.

Although women's access to work in small accommodation establishments is constrained by the honour–shame code, the growth of tourism has brought about alternative employment opportunities in hotels. The demand for labour within large hotels in Northern Cyprus tends to be gender-neutral as the hotels are operated according to an ethos of 'rational management'. Both men and women apply for the newly created jobs. The supply of female labour consists mainly of younger and more educated women who, on occasions, attain management level. Traditional gender norms are not entirely absent from large hotels but determine the specific occupations which it is appropriate for women and men to undertake. For example, it is not acceptable for Turkish Cypriot women to undertake waitressing or bar work. Thus, work in hotels generally falls within Purcell's category of contingently gendered jobs, in contrast to the patriarchally prescribed occupations which dominate the guesthouse sector.

Diversity within the female workforce in the accommodation sector is accompanied by a division of labour, by race, in the entertainment sector. For example, the demand for labour in casinos is met not by local Cypriot women but by women from East European countries. The work itself falls clearly within the category of sex-typed occupations and an alternative ideology of social sexuality is applied to the immigrant women who undertake it. Such racial divisions within the female workforce in Northern Cyprus have the effect of reinforcing traditional Cypriot norms concerning the limits of acceptable behaviour but, at the same time, facilitate Cypriot women's entry into other forms of tourism employment.

In contrast to the case of guesthouses in Northern Cyprus, Veronica Long and Sara Kindon show how homestays in Bali are managed by women, who engage in a wide range of social interactions with the tourists who stay in them. For example, Balinese women accompany tourists to the public forum of the local market. Women are also employees and managers in businesses producing silver and gold handicrafts, although their work in these enterprises is additional to their responsibility for domestic labour and childcare. More men than women manage tourist bungalows and restaurants and act as tour guides outside the boundaries of domestic activities.

Although employment in small tourism enterprises is structured by gender, Balinese women are not subject to the same patriarchal norms as those prevailing in Northern Cyprus. Women in Bali have access to a wider range of occupations in small enterprises and obtain significant additional earnings from their activities, higher status and a recognition of their business ability. However, the extent of their social interactions with tourists is determined by norms relating to sexuality and it is not acceptable for women to interact with tourists outside the confines of domestically related activities. Thus, for example, women are not employed in tourism transportation activities. Moreover, women experience a heavy workload and generally lack control over the allocation of household income to major expenditure items.

Racial divisions in the workforce come to the fore in the distribution of jobs within exclusive hotels, which are generally owned by outsiders. Higher paid and higher status occupations are the prerequisite of non-residents of Bali, who are subject to different social controls on their labour force participation. Labour force divisions also reflect diversity within the female Balinese workforce in that it is acceptable for unmarried women to work in some occupations in large hotels in the formal sector of the economy, whereas married women's labour supply is confined to small enterprises and the informal sector.

Social interactions between tourists and Balinese have increased awareness of different norms and values, providing scope for the renegotiation of culture (Picard, 1993). However, Long and Kindon argue that gender definitions in Bali are highly resistant to change. Although women's status has increased as the result of their tourism-related work, they have not experienced corresponding increases in their authority, power and control. Decision-making at levels higher than the household is undertaken by men, so that women lack power in the political hierarchy. Thus, Long and Kindon show that cultural preservation, which is sometimes said to be conducive to tourism, is inconsistent with gender equality.

The structuring of the tourism labour force in Mexico and the Philippines is, as elsewhere, predicated on women's major responsibility for domestic work and childcare, as Sylvia Chant shows. Women's work in the tourism industries of both countries has significant implications for their status, household structure and survival. Women obtain paid employment in hotels and restaurants and also work in the informal sector, selling such items as food and handicrafts. The income which they obtain is perceived as supplementing their husband's earnings and men generally maintain their dominant positions within the household. Within the Philippines, in particular, it is the duty of daughters to undertake domestic tasks and care for the family.

In Puerto Vallarta in Mexico, hotel managers demand women's labour for specific jobs, associated with prevailing gender norms. Thus, employment in hotels tends to be characterized by patriarchal capitalist relations, corresponding to Purcell's category of sex-typed occupations. The resulting segmentation in the structure of employment is legitimated not only by the association of women's paid work with their domestic responsibilities but also by managers' stated objective of minimizing sexual liaisons between men and women. The relative importance of women's employment as a share of total employment in hotels in Cebu in the Philippines is similar to that in Puerto Vallarta but the structure differs, as women's labour in Cebu is demanded for a wider range of occupations, including those which are not directly related to domestic tasks such as reception work in hotels. The nature of women's employment in non-administrative jobs in Mexican hotels reflects their major responsibility for domestic labour, whereas the differently segmented structure of employment in hotels in Cebu accords with the more equal participation of women and men in household work.

The accommodation sector in the Filipino town of Boracay consists of a higher proportion of small- and medium-sized enterprises than in Cebu, a lower degree of segmentation of the labour force and relatively more employment of women. Women generally work in housekeeping, laundrywork, administration and accounts and on the reception desk of hotels, and are only under-represented in gardening, maintenance, transportation and security. However, the gender division of labour in hotel restaurants differs from that of street-front restaurants. Within the latter industry, there is a higher demand for women to work as waitresses as it is assumed that women will attract more clients. Segmentation of work occurs in street and beach vending, where women and men supply different types of goods and services. Diversity also occurs within the female labour force as a greater percentage of young women work in the formal sector, in contingently gendered or sex-typed occupations, whereas older women tend to work in the informal sector.

The extreme form of sexuality based occupation in tourist destinations is, of course, prostitution, which is particularly prevalent in the Philippines and other South-East Asian destinations. As Urry (1990) observed, relations of racist as well as gender subordination underpin the demand for sex tourism in Asian countries. Many women supply their labour from a context of poverty, induced by relatively high material incentives or compelled by patriarchal networks between male household heads and local and national recruiters (Lee, 1991). Chant has shown how female prostitutes in the Philippines are often migrants from rural areas, many being single parents who attempt to cope with the pressures of their work by living with women friends or kin. Prostitution provides them with short-term employment while they are young and they subsequently attempt to find work in the informal sector.

The effects of women's work in the tourism industry vary between Mexico and the Philippines and between different occupations within each country. Although the opportunities for increased earnings and promotion are greater for men than for women in Mexico, women's earnings have enabled them to obtain more egalitarian relationships with men and, on occasions, to assert their independence from their male partners. They also use their earnings to educate both their sons and daughters and intend their daughters to achieve positions superior to their own. Women in the Philippines receive lower average earnings from their work in tourism than men and use their earnings to support their families. Unlike many Mexican women, they do not tend to leave their husbands even if they are unhappy in their relationships. They may use their savings to establish small businesses and, like Mexican women, generally obtain higher status from their work and associated income. The improvement in their material position, aided by their contact with women from other cultures, can provide them with an improved negotiating position within the household. However, both Mexican and Filipino women have a heavy workload and cannot always exercise control over expenditure from their earnings. Chant points out that segmentation of the labour force brings women together, providing scope for collective action. Collective action is, however, rare and alternative policy measures may be more effective in improving women's position, so long as they take account of women's roles in both paid work and the household.

Asian women's work is also examined by Muroi and Sasaki, in the context of prostitution tourism. Their analysis differs from the previous literature by identifying the changing material and ideological forces which have led to a partial shift of sex tourism from Asian destinations towards prostitution in the major origin country of Japan. Although the vast majority of Japanese tourists to Asian countries in past years have been men, women are increasing their demand for tourism. The material gains which tourist destinations can obtain from their expenditure provide an incentive for destinations to eliminate the most overt manifestations of sex tourism, as Leheny (1995) points out. On the other hand, ideological forces are also important. In particular, feminist groups in tourist origin and destination countries have coordinated campaigns to publicize sex tourism holidays. These have acted as an effective deterrent to sex tour provision by Japanese firms, in contrast to Leheny's view that changes in sex tour practices have only been cosmetic.

As the demand for prostitution tourism in Asian countries has declined, the commercialization of Asian women in Japan has increased. The demand for and supply of prostitution is historically embedded in Japanese culture and the subordinate position of Japanese women has led many to resign themselves to their husband's liaisons with prostitutes. Japanese women view their husband's relations with Asian prostitutes as a lesser threat to their own position than relations with Japanese prostitutes. Racial divisions between Japanese women and Asian women are compounded by vast disparities in income and wealth between Japan and such countries as Thailand and the Philippines. Thus, Muroi and Sasaki provide an answer to Leheny's question concerning the effects on Thai women of stricter controls on prostitution tourism in Thailand; not only is there a demand for Asian prostitutes in Japan but a supply of labour is forthcoming, as many Asian women lack income-generating opportunities in their own countries and accept the offer of work in the 'entertainment' sector of Japan.

Asian women's access to work in Japan is controlled by patriarchal relations as *Yakuza* syndicates form networks with local recruiters in order to 'import' Asian women into Japan, sometimes taking over the entire recruitment process. The women are often unaware of the work they will be undertaking and contract huge 'debts' as payment for their transportation to Japan. Once they are working as prostitutes in Japan, they have few or no alternative opportunities owing to their lack of knowledge of Japanese, lack of income and the social stigma which would be associated with returning to their families. Moreover, the earnings which they eventually obtain enable them to fulfil their expected role of caring for their families.

Asian women who work as prostitutes in Japan have pursued a range of strategies in response to the situations in which they find themselves. Many have accepted their assigned role in the absence of known alternatives or because they believe that this form of work can provide them and their families with a considerable improvement in living standards. Thai women are particularly vulnerable owing to their frequent status as illegal workers and fear that the Japanese authorities will take action against them. Some Asian women escape to refuges which have been established to aid prostitutes from overseas. A few have perceived no alternative but resort to violence, which has generally been directed against the most obvious target of the woman in charge of the establishment where they work; within their working situations, this appeared to be the only form of power and control which they could obtain. Legal measures which have been directed towards prostitution in Japan are unsatisfactory in that they confront the phenomenon of prostitution rather than its root causes and the conditions within which prostitutes work. Without a diminution of the disparities of wealth and power between industrialized and developing economies, and between men and women within them, there is little prospect of the disappearance of prostitution in destination or origin countries.

CONCLUSIONS

The rapidity with which the tourism industry has grown in recent years enables analyses of work in tourism to provide a range of insights into the processes by which labour markets are structured. Work in tourism forms a key locus of activity in destination countries, in contrast to the images of leisure which dominate tour operators' brochures. The tourism labour force in destination areas is clearly segmented by gender and race but what is also evident from the studies in this book is the variety of ways in which it is structured, both within and between countries. In Northern Cyprus, for example, patriarchal relations are particularly important in guest-houses, in contrast to the predominantly capitalist and 'patriarchal capitalist' production relations in hotels and casinos. In the UK, some hotels are characterized by capitalist relations of production, while patriarchal capitalist relations form the basis for work in some leisure parks and many public houses are managed according to patriarchal relations (Adkins, 1995). Capitalist relations involve gender neutrality in the demand for labour in the context of a gendered supply of labour. Patriarchal capitalist relations involve a gendered demand for labour, predicated on the prevailing gender-ing of the supply of labour. Patriarchal relations incorporate the key characteristic of control over women's labour, so that constraints on their access to work underlie the supply of and demand for labour. The different combinations of labour demand and supply give rise to Purcell's categories of contingently gendered jobs, sex-typed occu-pations and patriarchally prescribed occupations.

Prevailing norms of social sexuality impose limits on local women's contact with tourists and access to paid employment and public space in Northern Cyprus and Bali, while employment in hotels in Puerto Vallarta in Mexico is structured to limit social interactions between male and female employees. In contrast, British women are often expected to interact socially with male tourists as part of their jobs. Within the prostitution tourism and entertainment sectors of South-East Asia and Japan, sexual relations with tourists are commoditized, benefiting a range of intermediaries. In Cebu in the Philippines, employment is structured so that male workers can facilitate some guests' contacts with prostitutes, whereas in Boracay, women's sexuality is used to attract clients to restaurants in tourist-frequented streets.

It is clear that different types of production relations co-exist within the tourism industries of given economies and different combinations of production relations occur between economies. Hence, while generalized distinctions between capitalism and patri-archy may be of interest at the aggregate level, analysis at the micro level indicates the relevance of a range of theories of labour force segmentation which are not mutually exclusive. The applicability and relative importance of the different theories varies according to the diverse contexts and historical backgrounds of different countries and the material and ideological influences to which they have been subjected.

Consumers', employers' and workers' familiarity with different types of production, combined with the material interests which are implicit within them, means that particular types of production can persist in specific sectors over long periods. However, tourism can bring about some changes in the gender structuring of work. For example, expenditure by tourists may take the form of increased demand for accommodation in hotels in which the demand for labour tends to be gender-neutral or sex-typed rather than patriarchally prescribed. The greater availability of paid employment provides opportunities not only for men but for younger and more educated women, who may be less constrained in their social interactions with tourists than married women, as in the case of Northern Cyprus.

On the supply-side, ideologies of social sexuality impose constraints on the range of occupations which women undertake in tourism so that in Bali, for example, it is acceptable for women to manage accommodation establishments or shops but not to act as tour guides. In Northern Cyprus it is unacceptable for local women to work as croupiers in casinos so that these jobs have been undertaken by women from Russia and Rumania. None the less, the fact that some women transgress traditional norms of gender and social sexuality has the effect of extending the boundaries of acceptability in relation to local women's interactions with tourists and paid employment roles.

Social and political campaigns relating to working conditions also play a part in changing the nature of work in tourism and service activities. The internationally coordinated publicity campaigns which were organized to counter prostitution tourism are a case in point. Such campaigns can affect the location and conditions of work, particularly when supported by appropriate legal measures applying across countries; in the case of prostitution tourism, for example, public pressure has brought about some changes in the demand for prostitution. However, in the absence of significant material changes in those countries from which the supply of workers is forthcoming, the extent and effects of ideological changes tend to be limited.

By altering the demand for and supply of labour, tourism affects the relative earnings of men and women. Increased demand for workers to fill particular types of occupations increases men's or women's wages according to the gendering of labour demand. If constraints on women's labour supply are eased, average wages may fall, particularly if women are 'crowded' into specific occupations by a gendered demand for labour or by resistance to entry into alternative occupations on the part of male-dominated unions or bargaining associations. Thus, workers' associations may 'trade-off' an increased overall level of employment for the maintenance of higher wages for specific sectors of the labour force.

Tourism appears to have provided women, in particular, with increased opportunities for paid work and a higher level of earnings. Women's earnings are obtained both from employment in the formal sector and from such activities as selling food and handicrafts in the informal sector. Higher levels of disposable income resulting from participation in the tourism industry have benefited women in a number of ways, increasing their status and control over decision-making within the household, enabling them to choose alternative household relations and providing them with legitimate access to public space. However, such benefits have occurred within the context of an increased workload for women, a dominant ideology concerning the 'normal' heterosexual household structure, an unequal distribution of income within the household, unequal control over expenditure by household members and an absence of power and control over decision-making at community and higher levels. Thus, as Chant points out, strategies which aim to confront gender and race inequality should take account of both paid work and household relations.

The structuring of paid work on the basis of observable features of labour supply, notably sex and race, and the assignment of sets of gendered and race-based characteristics to them, masks the diversity of qualities and skills with which men and women are endowed. Explicit identification of the abilities which individuals possess or could develop would help to challenge traditional workforce divisions, including intra-occupational distinctions. It could also promote positive re-evaluation of specific gender and race-based characteristics. The latter process is under way in the field of marketing consumer goods, where retailers have become aware of the purchasing power of black consumers. Increased demand by tourists for more diverse work skills and qualities and a more equal gender and race balance in the workforce would not only bring about changes in the composition of labour demand; it would also provide a material underpinning for the re-evaluation of dominant gender and race definitions.

Dissatisfaction with many tourism 'products' which are currently being sold has led some researchers, consumers and pressure groups to call for alternative tourism. Within this context, demands for environmentally sustainable tourism have been prevalent. Such demands have sometimes been based on the premise that small-scale establishments are more conducive to environmental sustainability than large tourism organizations. Somewhat paradoxically, the establishment of large hotels, at times, provides more advantageous earnings and working conditions for previously disadvantaged groups than smaller enterprises which incorporate patriarchal relations of production. Hence, it is possible for demands for sustainability and alternative tourism to provide implicit support for traditional patterns of work and associated differences in status, power and rewards. It is, therefore, important for local, national and international programmes which propose to increase the number of tourism enterprises to identify not only the environmental sustainability of the projects under consideration but also the form of production relations and distribution of rewards which are incorporated within them.

It is clear that tourism-related work divisions vary both within and between societies so that no unique solution or programme is applicable to all societies and contexts. Tourism, *per se*, does not bring about a fundamental change in gender and race definitions and the structuring of work. Indeed, it frequently reinforces existing structures and work divisions. None the less, it provides an international context in which there is scope for change.

REFERENCES

Adkins, L. (1995) *Gendered Work. Sexuality, Family and the Labour Market*, Milton Keynes and Philadelphia: Open University Press.

Buck, R. (1977) 'The ubiquitous tourist brochure: explorations in its intended and unintended use', *Annals of Tourism Research*, 4(4): 192–207.

Cohen, C. Ballerino (1995) 'Marketing paradise, making nation', *Annals of Tourism Research*, 22(2): 404–21.

Davidson, D. (1985) 'Women in Thailand', *Canadian Women's Studies*, 16(1): 16–19.

Dilley, R.S. (1986) 'Tourist brochures and tourist images', *Canadian Geographer*, 30(1): 59–65.

Edensor, T. and Kothari, U. (1994) 'The masculinization of Stirling's heritage', in V. Kinnaird and D. Hall (eds) *Tourism: A Gender Analysis*, Chichester: Wiley.

Enloe, C. (1989) *Bananas, Beaches and Bases: Making Feminist Sense of International Politics*, London: Pandora.

Kinnaird, V. and Hall, D. (eds) (1994) *Tourism: A Gender Analysis*, Chichester: Wiley.

Lee, W. (1991) 'Prostitution and tourism in South-East Asia', in N. Redclift and M.T. Sinclair (eds) *Working Women. International Perspectives on Labour and Gender Ideology*, London and New York: Routledge.

Leheny, D. (1995) 'A political economy of Asian sex tourism', *Annals of Tourism Research*, 22(2): 441–62.

Momsen, J. Henshall (1994) 'Tourism, gender and development in the Caribbean', in V. Kinnaird and D. Hall (eds) *Tourism: A Gender Analysis*, Chichester: Wiley.

Picard, M. (1993) 'Cultural tourism in Bali: national integration and regional differentiation', in M. Hitchcock, V.T. King and M.G. Parnwell (eds) *Tourism in South-East Asia*, London and New York: Routledge.

Ramazanoglu, C. (1989) *Feminism and the Contradictions of Oppression*, London and New York: Routledge.

Smith, D. (1987) *The Everyday World as Problematic*, Milton Keynes: Open University Press.

Swain, M. Byrne (ed.) (1995) *Gender in Tourism*, special issue of *Annals of Tourism Research*, 22(2).

Urry, J. (1990) *The Tourist Gaze: Leisure and Travel in Contemporary Societies*, London: Sage.

Index

accommodation and catering 123–4; agro-tourism 4; bed and breakfast 112; family-owned hotels 74–6, 77–8, 80; homestays 99–102, 107, 109; institutionally owned hotels 74, 80, 81–4; premises 77–8; women workers 36–7, 39–40

Acker, J. 7

Adkins, L. 5, 7, 8, 45–6, 47, 48, 49–50, 155, 223, 230

Adorno, T. 24

advertising holidays: black people 21, 24; brochures 17–24; objectification of women 16, 19–21; sexual sell 21–2

aesthetic, gendered 29–31

agro-tourism 4

Aguilar, D. 128, 130, 133

Airtours brochure 18

Aldana, C. 133

alternative tourism 61, 233

Angeles, L. 130

Ariani, G. 96, 97

Ariani, I. G. A. 102, 103

Arias, P. 131

Arizmendi, F. 131

Arizpe, L. 134

Arjani, L. 97

Armstrong, K. 61, 109

art shops 104, 105

Asahi Shimbun 191

Ashton, S. 63

Asia, South-East: Japanese tourists 185–6; prostitution tourism 181–2, 183–4, 188, 190–1, 228; women's diversity 201–7; see also individual countries

Asian Development Bank 183

Asian Women's Association 205

Asian Women's Shelter HELP 202, 205

Awanohara, S. 181

Azarcon de la Cruz, P. 134, 145

Bacon, W. 38

Badger, A. 46

Bagguley, P. 4, 39

Bali: airport 92; culture 92, 94, 99; day cruises 104–5, 107; decision making 97–8; economic autonomy of women 98; entrepreneurship, local/foreign 112; exclusive hotels 105–6, 107; family homestays 99–102, 107, 109; gender ideology 91–8, 106–11; low-budget tourists 92; shops for tourists 102–3, 105–6, 107; socio-cultural system 95–6; surfer bungalows 104–5, 107; tourism development 91–4, 114; tourism employment 105, 106–13, 225; Women in Development 97, 98

Bali Sustainable Development Project 98–9

Barry, K. 5

Barry, T. 123